Acta Neurochirurgica
Supplements

Editor: H.-J. Reulen
Assistant Editor: H.-J. Steiger

SpringerWienNewYork

Training in Neurosurgery

Proceedings of the
Conference on Neurosurgical Training and Research
Munich, October 6–9, 1996

Edited by
H.-J. Reulen and H.-J. Steiger

Acta Neurochirurgica
Supplement 69

SpringerWienNewYork

Prof. Dr. Hans-Jürgen Reulen
Prof. Dr. Hans-Jakob Steiger
Neurochirurgische Universitätsklinik, Klinikum Großhadern, München,
Federal Republic of Germany

ISBN-13: 978-3-7091-7419-7   e-ISBN-13: 978-3-7091-6860-8
DOI: 10.1007/978-3-7091-6860-8

© 1997 Springer-Verlag/Wien
Softcover reprint of the hardcover 1st edition 1997

Typesetting: Best-Set Typesetter Ltd., Hong Kong
Printing: A. Holzhausens Nfg., A–1070 Wien
Graphic design: Ecke Bonk

Printed on acid-free and chlorine free bleached paper
SPIN: 10630873

With 29 Figures

ISSN 0065-1419
ISBN-13: 978-3-7091-7419-7 Springer-Verlag Wien New York

Preface

An applicant accepted in the year 1997 for a neurosurgical residency program will have finished his residency at the earliest in 2003. In fact, we have to consider that we are now training the neurosurgeons for the first 3 decades of the 21st century. Are we sure that our training program does meet the needs of the future? Do we convey the necessary theoretical and practical background to educate competent and respected clinicians and surgeons, innovative investigators, and stimulating instructors and teachers? Will our residents be prepared to cope with the explosion of new information in neuroscience, the health care reforms, the political pressures of socioeconomic changes, etc. in these turbulent times? Is our speciality prepared to successfully deal with these challenges? Very much is depending on whether we continue to remain attractive to bright, very talented and highly motivated young people, the best of the medical school graduates. They will only be attracted if we can convincingly demonstrate that neurosurgery is a most promising and rewarding speciality and that they will receive the best possible training.

The present and future teachers have the responsibility to create the necessary environment for the best possible training. But we all are aware that the individual teacher cannot solve all the many problems involved in creating a modern training program. It needs our readiness for a common effort. We have to agree on a structured curriculum, we have to define our desired standards, we have to accept regular quality reviewing of our programs according to some formal requirements. We also need to include modern teaching techniques. If we are not providing the standards ourselves, public and legal pressures will eventually demand to ensure them.

It is a good time to start the exciting task of re-structuring neurosurgical training. Education is also a rewarding task, as many of our successful and highly estimated teachers experienced in the past. Our trainees will be thankful lifelong and pass on this spirit further.

An International Conference on *"Neurosurgical Training and Research"* was held in Munich from October 6–9, 1996, under the auspices of the EANS (European Association of Neurological Societies), and organized by H.-J. Reulen and H.-J. Steiger. The idea was to have experts from various countries and neurosurgical organizations collect information on the present status of resident training in our speciality and the mechanisms involved with the training. Various aspects, the recruitment process, the criteria used for selection, the contents and structure of a program, the continuous quality control, exposition to the art of research, fellowships and subspeciality training, etc. have been covered. The present book contains this material and thus provides a unique and comprehensive source of information on the complex of modern neurosurgical training.

We extend our compliments to Mario Brock and Luc Calliauw who helped us prepare the Conference; we have to thank the members of the Advisory Board, A. Baethman, R. Braakman, D. Long, J. D. Miller†; K. Takakura, N. de Tribolet, and we are particularly grateful to all authors who prepared their manuscripts in time to meet our deadline. We also wish to acknowledge our gratitude to Springer Verlag, Vienna, for the technical support and for the prompt publication of this volume.

Munich, May 1997

H.-J. Reulen
H.-J. Steiger

Contents

National Mechanisms for the Selection of Neurosurgical Trainees

Pevehouse, B. C.: Matching Program for Appointment to Residency Training in Neurological Surgery in United States   1
Hide, T. A. H.: National Mechanisms for the Selection of Trainees. Procedure in Great Britain   6

Criteria to Find Qualified Candidates

Brock, M.: Leadership Qualities in Prominent Neurosurgeons   8
Gilsbach, J. M., Pillong, A.: Criteria to Find Qualified Candidates – Professional Personnel Recruitment Methods Adapted to Neurosurgery   12
Kohlhofer, I.: Criteria and Procedures in the Automotive Industry   19
Jarosch, H.-W.: Selection of Air Force Officers – Profiles, Criteria, Testing   22
Neil-Dwyer, G., Lang, D. A.: Can We Define or Measure Manual Skills in Surgical Training?   27

How Many Residents Shall We Train?

Patterson Jr., R. H.: How many Residents Should we Train? The USA Experience   30
Tulleken, C. A. F.: How many Residents Shall we Train? The Netherlands Experience   33
Shaw, M. D. M.: How Many Higher Neurosurgical Trainees Shall We Train in the British Isles?   36
Gjerris, F., Madsen F. F.: How Many Neurosurgeons Do We Want to Educate in Europe Annually? The Danish Proposal   40
Lobo Antunes, J.: How Many Residents Shall We Train? The Iberian Experience   43
Cohadon, F.: Neurosurgical Manpower in France   45
Schramm, J.: How Many Residents Shall We Train – The Situation In Germany   47
Takakura, K.: How Many Neurosurgeons Should We Train? The Japanese Experience   55

Contents and Structure of a Training Program

Long, D. M.: Neurosurgical Training at Present and in the Next Century   58
Calliauw, L.: The UEMS Model – Proposals for Classification and Training Durations of Specialties Registered in Doctors' Directives   65
Yoshimoto, T., Tominaga, T.: Contents and Structure of a Training Program. The Japanese Proposal   70
Pendl, G.: Neurosurgical Training in Austria – Present Status and Aspects for the Future   73
Cabiol, J.: A Resident's Experience and Suggestion   75
Haase, J.: Control and Structure of a Training Program. The View of a Non-academic Hospital   79

Assessment of Training Progress and Examinations

Hoff, J. T., Eisenberg, H. M.: Assessment of Training Progress and Examinations   83
Braakman, R.: Experience with the EANS Examinations   89
Pickard, J. D.: Experience with the United Kingdom Examinations in Neurosurgery   93
Vapalahti, M.: Periodic Evaluation of Training Progress and Teaching   98
Schramm, J.: What Consequences Should Result from Failure to Meet Internal Standards?   101

Research and Research Training

Reulen, H.-J.: When Should Residents be Exposed to Research? 106
Meßmer, K., Baethmann, A.: Role of Surgical Research in the Training of Neurosurgeons 111
Teasdale, G. M.: Research in Neurosurgical Training: Clinical Reviews and Trials 116
Fahlbusch, R.: From the Scientific Idea to its Realisation – Principles and Strategies in Neurosurgery 120

Fellowship and Subspeciality Training

Ostertag, Ch.: Subspeciality Training in Neurosurgery 126
Sonntag, V. K. H.: Neurosurgical Spine Fellowships: The Phoenix Model 130
Raimondi, A. J.: A Model Fellowship in Pediatric Neurosurgery 135
Piepgras, D. G.: Post Residency Subspecialty Training in Neurosurgery – The Impact of Subspecialty
    Training on Organized Neurosurgery and Resident Training – Benefits, Responsibilities and Liabilities 140

Neurosurgical Training of the Future

Apuzzo, M. L. J.: In The Realm of Ideas: the Advent of Advanced Surgery of the Human Cerebrum and
    Neurosurgical Education 145
Buess, G.: The Development of Training Systems in General Surgery 151
Batschkus, M. M.: Interactive Multimedia Software for Training and Education in Neurosurgery 156

Index of Keywords 159

Listed in Current Contents

Acta Neurochir (1997) [Suppl] 69:1–5

Matching Program for Appointment to Residency Training in Neurological Surgery in United States

B. C. Pevehouse

Department of Neurosurgery, University of California Medical Center, San Francisco, CA, U.S.A.

Keywords: Matching program, residency training, selection process.

In the late 1920's, the American Medical Association evolved a process of identifying and approving postgraduate medical education in the United States. The first record of formal residency training in neurological surgery appeared in the AMA Directory in September, 1933, offering one position at the Medical College of Virginia in Richmond. Over the subsequent years and particularly after World War II, residency training programs were developed throughout the country, with a peak number of 194 by 1965, 55 of which were not affiliated with a medical school and provided little more than a personal preceptorship with the director. At this time, a Residency Review Committee was established to review training programs and to set minimum standards for accreditation. By 1983, the number of programs was reduced to 94, offering about 130 first year positions each year for a term of five or more years of tightly structured residency training. Appointments were made individually by each program director, sometimes years in advance for outstanding candidates, but each year some positions would be unfilled and directors would complain about the scarcity of qualified applicants.

Thus in 1983, The Society of Neurological Surgeons approved the National Neurological Surgery Matching Program (NSMP) for first year (postgraduate year 2) neurosurgical residency training for appointments beginning in July 1985. All directors of United States neurosurgical residency training programs agreed to participate and abide by the rules of the Match, designed to make the process fair for both applicant and director. Neither the applicant nor the program director may ask for a commitment before the Match. Directors agree not to offer or to make any appointments before the Match. All ranking lists are confidential. Both parties are bound by the results of the Match. It is a secret ballot of free choice creating an auction for the highest bidder for all positions simultaneously; thus, there is no leverage, no coercion to make an immediate decision, and no uncertainty that one might wait too long to make a decision and thus lose the first choice. If an applicant receives several offers in the process, the applicant will match to the program that is highest on his or her list. If several applicants want the same training program, the program will get the applicant(s) who are highest on its list. A few positions may remain unfilled and unmatched applicants then negotiate on their own for the rare unfilled positions. The NSMP coordinator provides a vacancy telephone "hotline" to facilitate this process after the Match is completed and maintained throughout the year to advise any callers of available positions created by residents leaving training.

The Matching Process

I will describe the details and timetable of the next Match, which is scheduled for January 13, 1997, for appointments beginning in July, 1998. In May 1996, Program Announcements, including a registration form and letter describing the specialty and required training, are distributed to the Deans of U. S. medical schools and to the residency program directors (Appendix 1, pages a–g).

Table 1. *Matching Program for Appointment to Residency Training in Neurological Surgery (United States Programs)*

	10 Year Average 1985-94	Beginning Residency July 1995	Beginning Residency July 1996	Beginning Residency July 1997
Number of PGY-2 Positions Listed in Directory (1st year residency in neurological surgery)	134	145	146	148
Number of Residency Programs	93	97	97	97
Total Positions Offered in Match	131	141	141	140
Number of Registrants	387	425	479	460
Number Submitting Ranking List	246	251	276	258
Positions Filled by Match	129	139	141	140
Positions Unfilled in Match (filled from pool of unmatched applicants within a few days)	2	2	0	0
Applicants Who Received Offer But Did Not List That Program and Were Not Matched	5	1	4	2
Number of Applicants Not Matched	116	112	135	118
Number of Applicants Not Listed By Any Program	28	30	20	26
IMGs Submitting Ranking List	30	34	51	31
IMGs Matched	4	7	7	3

Table 2. *Matching Program for Residency in Neurological Surgery*

Match in January 1995 for Training Beginning July 1, 1996
Applicants: 238 applicants reported 6,378 applications = 26.8 per applicant
229 applicants reported 2,098 interviews = 9.2 per applicant
276 applicants ranked 2,368 programs, an average of 8.6 per rank list

The 141 matched applicants obtained a rank list choice of

Choice	Number of applicants
1st	53
2nd	19
3rd	13
4th	8
5th	9
6–10th	31
11–15th	7
16–20th	1

The interested candidate completes the registration form and submits it with a fee of $35 to the NSMP office in San Francisco. The registrant receives a Directory of all neurosurgical residency programs and instructions on making formal application for appointment by submitting a ranking list of preferred residency programs and by signing a binding agreement to accept a Match offer.

After registration, applicants make specific application to and visit selected programs, serve clinical clerkships, arrange for interviews and decide if neurological surgery is their career choice, as well as deciding which programs are most desirable for their own training. Directors prepare their ranking list of acceptable applicants. Programs and applicants submit their rank-ordered preference lists to the NSMP office by January 13, 1997. After all lists are received and errors/omissions corrected (often requiring personal telephone calls by the coordinator), the Match is conducted and results telefaxed to the office of the respective medical school Dean and to

Table 3. *Matching Program for Residency in Neurological Surgery*

Match in January 1995 for Training Beginning July 1, 1996
Residency Programs: 92 programs offered and filled 141 positions

For all 141 positions in all 92 programs, this rank choice was obtained:

Choice	Number of applicants
1st	28
2nd	23
3rd	13
4th	20
5th	12
6th	12
7th	13
8th	9
9th	3
10th	3
11th	2
12th	1
13th	1
19th	1

Table 4. *Matching Program for Residency in Neurological Surgery*

Match in January 1995 for Training Beginning July 1, 1996
Residency Programs: 92 programs offered and filled 141
  positions

The first position in each program was filled by this rank choice:

Choice	Number of applicants
1st	28
2nd	19
3rd	6
4th	11
5th	8
6th	7
7th	7
8th	2
9th	2
10th	2

the program director, with confirmation by mail to all applicants.

We now have thirteen years' experience with this annual process. Recent review indicates full acceptance by both applicants and program directors and a highly successful process and outcome, satisfactory for everyone except for the qualified applicants who failed to obtain a residency position. The ratio of applicants to available positions has been almost 2:1 each year (Table 1).

Detailed analysis of the first eleven years of the Match was published in 1994 [1]. The study revealed that 3,954 applications and ranking lists were received; 729 were repeated applications by unmatched applicants in one or more subsequent years, thus there was a net total of 3,225 applicants, of which 1,455 were matched for appointment into neurosurgical residency training.

How successful is the selection and matching process for the individual applicant or program director? Analysis of the January 1995 Match notes that 53/141 applicants obtained their first choice program and 85/141 were in the top 3 ranking (Table 2); programs had a more even distribution of matched choices, yet 96/141 positions were matched to top 5 ranking (Table 3); and 28 matched applicants were the program's first choice (Table 4).

Careful review of the published 1994 study will provide many details concerning the Match [1]. For example, that 15 matched applicants did not commence residency training in neurological surgery, 157 residents did not complete training, and 42 residents

transferred to a different program before completing training.

The Match offers advantages to both applicants and program directors. By creating a set calendar and a more orderly and visible process, all concerned parties know what and when certain actions are required. Also the programs that did not fill all positions in the Match are known, affording those qualified individuals who did not match, either through misperception of their abilities, poor advice, or the luck of the draw, an opportunity to a find a position for neurosurgical training. Lastly, but still important, neurosurgical educators can determine the number of serious applicants seeking neurosurgical training each year.

Appendix

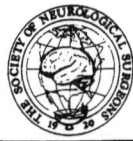

NEUROLOGICAL SURGERY MATCHING PROGRAM

Sponsored by The Society of Neurological Surgeons

PROGRAM ANNOUNCEMENT

The Society of Neurological Surgeons announces the following services for applicants interested in a career in Neurological Surgery.

PGY-2 MATCH for NEUROLOGICAL SURGERY

The next Neurological Surgery Match will take place on **January 13, 1997.** *See timetable.*
This match will be for applicants who wish to start their PGY-2 in July, 1998.

Registration: Complete and mail the attached form as soon as possible. Extra forms are available from your Neurological Surgery department, Dean's office or from NSMP.

Fee: The $35 fee is non-refundable and covers registration and matching

Deadline: Applicant and program ranking lists must reach our office on or before January 13, 1997. *See timetable.*

Results: On January 20 results will be available at your Dean's office. On that day, letters are mailed to each applicant.

VACANCY INFORMATION SYSTEM

Vacancies for 1996 or 1997 positions, submitted by program directors, will be announced on the Vacancy Information System.
CALL 1-415-923-3907
(a free service, available day and night)

NEUROLOGICAL SURGERY
MATCHING PROGRAM
1996 TIMETABLE

Early 1996 — Gather information about Neurological Surgery as a career choice. Register with NSMP on the attached form. You will receive the Directory of participating programs.

Summer 1996 — Send your applications to training programs and plan your interviews. It is your responsibility to arrange these interviews.

Fall 1996 — Some training programs will accept applications at any time; others may set a deadline. Interviews may start.

November 1996 — Release of Dean's letters. Interviews will continue. Also plan PGY-1 interviews.

January 1997 — Programs and applicants submit their rank-ordered preference lists to NSMP. All forms must be received at NSMP on or before the NSMP deadline.

January 13, 1997	**Deadline, Matching starts**
January 20, 1997	**Match Results** are FAXed to your Dean's office and mailed to you
February 21	NRMP deadline for PGY-1
March 19	PGY-1 results known

The timetable is tight; therefore, you should consider interviewing for PGY-1 positions and for alternate choices (in case you do not match in Neurological Surgery) before the NSMP match.

June, 1997	PGY-1 starts
July, 1998	Neurosurgery training starts

Page b

How It Works

All training programs will submit rank-ordered lists of the applicants they would like to accept into their program. The applicants will submit rank-ordered lists of programs they want to go to. *All ranking lists are strictly confidential.*

This year, our match procedures have been modified in response to the concerns many applicants had about matching algorithms. Although there is only a 0.1% chance that the results of the old algorithm would differ from the revised one, the new algorithm ensures that applicants' preferences will *always* prevail. Through the matching process, we will first seek to place you in the program at the top of your list. If that program has more applicants than positions, its lower ranked placement requests will be denied. If this happens to you, your request will be passed to the next program on your list, and so on.

This procedure guarantees that you will be matched to the first program on your list that accepts you. The outcome of the match has no elements of chance and is determined solely by the confidential ranking lists. A more extensive description of the process is included in the NSMP Directory.

Registration and Matching Fee

With your request for registration, you must submit a $35.00 non-refundable fee. There is no additional fee for the actual match. Programs also pay a fee.

Training Requirements

Before entering a Neurological Surgery training program, you must have completed a 12-month internship (including at least 6 months of surgery). For residents starting in July, 1997 this will usually be an internship obtained through the February, 1996 NRMP match. The director of the program to which you have been matched may assist you in obtaining an internship.

To be eligible for certification by the American Board of Neurological Surgery, you must have completed your PGY-1 year and five years in an accredited Neurological Surgery residency program. The oral part of the Board examination can be taken after two years of practice.

Page c

Interviews

It is your responsibility to contact each program you are interested in, to ask for detailed information and to follow each program's application and interview procedures. *Consult the timetable for dates.*

You should know that you are under no obligation to reveal your program preferences and that participating programs cannot make you a binding offer other than through the matching program. Both parties are free to change their intention, without prejudice, up to the time the final, confidential rank-order lists are submitted.

Match Results Are Binding

The match results constitute a **binding commitment** from which neither the applicant nor the program director can withdraw without mutual agreement.

After the match, unfilled positions can be negotiated directly by uncommitted applicants. Previously matched applicants are NOT eligible to apply for other positions unless they provide written evidence that they have been released from their obligation.

Previous Matching Programs

The first Neurological Surgery Matching Program took place in 1983; presently, all civilian training programs participate. In the 1996 match, 276 applicants competed to fill 141 positions. Of the participating U.S. seniors, 72% matched; of those matched, 67% obtained one of their top three choices.

Vacancy Information System

Vacancies for PGY-2 positions in 1996 and 1997, when submitted by program directors, will be announced in frequently updated telephone recordings which can be reached by calling our main number:

1-415-923-3907

Applicants and program directors are free to negotiate these positions individually. Any positions remaining unfilled after the next match will also be listed.

For further information and for discussion of special circumstances, please contact the NSMP Office.

August Colenbrander, M.D., Coordinator
P.O. Box 7999
San Francisco, CA 94120-7999
1-415-923-3907

Page d

NEUROLOGICAL SURGERY
MATCHING PROGRAM
REQUEST FOR REGISTRATION

Please register me for the January 19____ Matching Program and send me the Directory of participating programs.

First name: _____ Middle initial: _____

Last name: _____

Address: _____

_____

City: _____

State: _____ Zip: _____

Medical School: _____
(indicate country, if not U.S.A.)

Year of graduation: _____

Please provide a telephone number (not necessarily your own) where we can reliably reach you, if necessary, during the matching period.

(____)_____ Relationship: _____

[ ] My non-refundable check for $35 is enclosed, payable to:

Neurological Surgery Matching Program
P.O. Box 7999
San Francisco, CA 94120-7999

[ ] Please charge my fee to my Visa / MasterCard:

____ ____ ____ ____

Expiration date: __ / __

Date: _____ Signature: _____

Page e

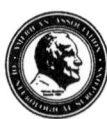 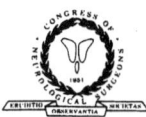 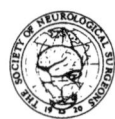

April 1996

Dear Third Year Medical Student:

Residency positions in Neurological Surgery are assigned through the Neurological Surgery Matching Program. The purpose of this letter is to provide you with a brief overview of the specialty of Neurosurgery to aid you in your career decision.

In essence, Neurological Surgery is concerned with the diagnosis and treatment, usually surgical, of disorders involving the central, peripheral, or autonomic nervous systems. This is a system-based, rather than regional, discipline, a fact that adds to the excitement and continuing challenge of the specialty. An active neurological surgeon may, in the course of a single day, find himself evacuating a blood clot from the brain, removing a ruptured disc from the lumbar spinal canal, and transposing a compressed ulnar nerve anterior to the elbow joint. All this in addition to consulting on patients referred to his office or in hospital, interpreting specialized radiological studies such as CT scans, magnetic resonance images and angiograms, and visiting with pre- and post-operative patients in the hospital.

The practice of Neurological Surgery is concerned with all age groups. A meningomyelocele may require closure within a few hours after birth. A newborn with an enlarging head may need diagnostic studies, subdural aspirations, or shunting procedures for hydrocephalus within the first weeks of life. Children may present with brain and spinal cord tumors and vascular malformations of the nervous system. Adults suffer from disc disease, usually in the lumbar and cervical regions, primary and metastatic brain tumors, aneurysms of cerebral blood vessels, and occlusive disease of the extracranial blood vessels supplying the brain. Trauma to the central and peripheral nervous systems is unfortunately widespread and not linked to specific age groups. Infants suffer birth injuries, fall, and are occasionally subjected to abuse at home. Teenagers are involved in vehicular accidents. Working people experience traumatic incidents at their jobs, and the elderly are prone to falls or violence with resultant skull and spinal fractures as well as blood clots compressing adjacent nervous structures.

Neurological Surgery is a relatively new discipline, dating back to the early part of this century. From its beginnings the specialty has been wedded firmly to the laboratory. The founders and pathfinders in Neurosurgery: Sir Victor Horsley; Harvey Cushing; Walter Dandy; Wilder Penfield; and many others, while all technically skillful surgeons, were, in many respects, clinical neurophysiologists. During their careers they shuttled between their experimental laboratories, clinical wards, and operating theaters seeing problems, asking questions, and designing appropriate investigative tactics for their resolution. This tradition of a discipline whose practitioners are intellectually restless and rarely satisfied with old maxims or current statistics holds true to the present time. Most neurosurgical residency programs offer, and many require, time to be spent in the laboratory working on a variety of problems and acquiring certain specialized skills. Today's investigative techniques are sophisticated, expensive, and the skills often take years to master. Each year it becomes increasingly more difficult for even a very talented individual to be both a first-class investigator and a top-flight neurosurgeon. Nonetheless, to be satisfied with our present body of knowledge and our current techniques is both intellectually unrewarding and constitutes a certain pathway to obsolescence. In the future we will continue to recruit and train individuals who can recognize clinical problems that demand solutions, pose the appropriate questions, help in the planning of laboratory experiments, and will be able to evaluate and interpret the resultant data.

A few statistics: Neurological Surgery is a relatively small specialty with approximately 3,300 Board-certified practitioners, constituting about 0.7% of the physicians in the United States. There are approximately 94 approved training programs in the United States and Canada, virtually all associated with a medical school. About 130 residents finish training each year with about 140 entering the training cycle each July. Approximately 700 residents are in training at any particular time. The minimum training period is five years after at least one year of postgraduate training in general surgery, some programs require six years after your PGY-1.

For those of you who are seriously considering Neurological Surgery as a possible career and wish to apply for the Neurosurgical Residency Matching Program, we would recommend perusal of the Special Article published by the Journal, *NEUROSURGERY*. (Vol. 35:1172-1182, December, 1994). This ar ticle provides details about the application process and matching program each year for acceptance into a U.S. approved program for residency training in neurological surgery. Information concerning specific training programs in the Directory you receive upon registration.

Several things should be apparent at this juncture. Neurological Surgery is a demanding specialty by many criteria: hours expended, physical stamina required, and emotional toll extracted. The training period is long, and there are only a limited number of slots available. Furthermore, there are very few opportunities for "midcourse" career corrections once one has become fully engaged in neurosurgical practice. Why then should you, as a third-year medical student, consider this specialty as a possible career choice?

The answer is complex, involving a melange of intellectual, personal, and emotional considerations. Obviously, the specialty appeals to someone who is intrigued by a need to understand how the human brain -- that most complicated of all computers -- both functions and malfunctions. There are few intellectual challenges more satisfying than pinpointing a pathological lesion within the nervous system on the basis of a detailed history and meticulous neurological examination. To be able to verify one's putative clinical impression by precise neuroradiological imaging procedures and then confirm the diagnosis at operation is a soul-satisfying exercise.

But Neurosurgery involves much more than an intellectual challenge. Neurosurgeons are interventionists, willing to make decisions and accept responsibilities involving not only life and death but encompassing those vital functions of the brain and spinal cord such as movement, sensation, vision, speech, intellect, and emotion. In brief, the entire fabric of what distinguishes a sentient functioning human being. One must possess the humanity to relate and communicate honestly with patients and their families under conditions of extreme stress, the humility and sense of proportion to comprehend what is attainable and what is beyond reach, and, most importantly, the sense of one's own self to combat the despair and self-doubt that inevitably creep in when one's best efforts fall short of expectations.

This is a challenging, demanding, exciting discipline whose intellectual and technical frontiers are being expanded at an almost incomprehensible pace. There will never be a great demand for a multitude of neurosurgeons but, like certain elite military units, we will always need a select few who will feel unfulfilled as physicians and human beings if they are not pushed to the limits of their capabilities. Most neurosurgeons in practice today would, even in retrospect, make the same choice they did many years ago.

Neurological Surgery, for all its difficulties, when done well, not only gives one a great sense of personal satisfaction but is capable of making great differences in the lives of our patients.

Good luck in your choice of a medical career.

Byron C. Pevehouse, M.D.

Chairman, Advisory Committee on the Neurological Surgery Matching Program, for The Society of Neurological Surgeons

Page g

Page f

References

1. Pevehouse B, Colenbrander A (1994) The United States Neurological Surgery Residency Matching Program. Neurosurgery 35: 1172–1182
2. Pevehouse B, Siegel G (1996) 1995 Comprehensive neuro-surgical practice survey. American Association of Neurological Surgeons, Park Ridge, IL

Correspondence: Prof. Dr. B. C. Pevehouse, University of California Medical Center, Department of Neurological Surgery, 94143 San Francisco, CA, U.S.A.

Acta Neurochir (1997) [Suppl] 69:6–7

National Mechanisms for the Selection of Trainees. Procedure in Great Britain

T. A. H. Hide

Southern General Hospital, Glasgow, United Kingdom

Keywords: Selection of Trainees, Procedure in Great Britain.

Selection for and career progression in medicine and surgery in the United Kingdom and Ireland are broadly similar. After completing school and university, a pre-registration year is spent as *Junior House Officer* usually with six months in medicine and six months in surgery. Following this, the aspirant to surgical training will apply for a basic surgical training post (*Senior House Officer*). This is for a minimum of two years but may be extended to three after which the trainee will sit an examination of one of the Royal Colleges to obtain a Membership of the Royal College of Surgeons (MRCS). The next stage in training is to obtain a higher surgical training post in the grade of *Specialist Registrar*. This will be in the specific surgical specialty in which the trainee wishes to become qualified and lasts for a period of six years in which there will be organised periods for research and travel, most often towards the end of the training period.

There is therefore no specific selection to enter neurosurgical training except in the competitive situation of obtaining a higher surgical training post in neurosurgery. The number of such posts is quite rigidly limited by agreement between the profession and the Department of Health. After the fourth year in this training programme, the trainee can sit the Intercollegiate Examination in Neurosurgery and if successful will obtain a Fellowship of the Royal College of Surgeons in that specialty (FRCS Surgical Neurology).

In order to be placed on the European Specialist Register, a trainee must have completed the six years of higher surgical training successfully and hold the FRCS in the specialty. As from 1997 only those trainees who have been placed on the Specialist Register can gain appointment to a Consultant Neurosurgical post in the Health Service. This is a post of full autonomous responsibility for the care of patients.

While there is no specific selection for neurosurgery, this highly pyramidal structure of career progression together with intense competition for the limited number of university places and training posts ensures a high general level of competence and ability in the trainees selected for neurosurgical training.

In Great Britain, selection for Neurosurgery is both internal and external as in many other countries. Internal selection can be influenced by many factors. Exposure to the specialty through friends and relatives, personal experience and even novels and the media may provoke and interest. Occasionally, this can become obsessional and this has to be carefully guarded against in selection but occasionally can result in high motivation.

External selection for all medical training is in some ways worryingly dependent on academic ability rather than seeking evidence in the candidates of characteristics and skills which may specifically equip them for a career in Neurosurgery.

The actual selection into higher surgical training in neurosurgery is done by a selection committee which comprises Neurosurgeons, both academic and non-academic, specialists from other disciplines, external assessors from outwith the appointing Unit and is chaired by a lay person. While the candidates may be previously known to some of those in the Committee, the interview itself rarely lasts longer than one hour and is not supported by any form of psychological profiling or aptitude testing.

It would not be unreasonable to characterise selection for neurosurgery in the United Kingdom and Ireland at present as intuitive, amateurish, very personally based and potentially wasteful. It is however highly competitive and especially in a small specialty like neurosurgery where there are only about 160 Consultant Neurosurgeons, can be quite constant in the unwritten criteria used.

Most certainly, it does not even approach the detailed and complex selection process used by many industrial and financial business concerns.

In some ways, it has become a "trial by committee"! While this most certainly requires high performance under stress, it tends to favour the eloquent, somewhat extroverted person at the expense of the more introverted academic yet highly motivated and sometimes more manually dextrous candidate. More seriously, it favours the native English speaker and does limit the opportunities for non-residents to obtain full neurosurgical training in Britain.

Due to a lack of objective criteria, the British system has the disadvantage of

- Tending to discriminate against women and minority ethnic groups.
- Leads to accusations of unfairness from those rejected.
- May select those with persistence and lack of insight rather than those with true talent and ability.

It does however, have the advantages of

- Allowing non-conformists to enter neurosurgical training.
- Allowing several "trys" to obtain a training post helping to cancel out obstruction by personal animosity and bias.
- Allows selection of candidates on non-medical criteria enabling them to bring useful and important non-medical skills and experience into neurosurgery.

It seems clear that we do need to have a better structured selection process in the United Kingdom and Ireland. This is not only to maintain standards and safeguard the public but also to avoid waste. The inappropriate use and placement of that most scarce of resources – intelligent, highly motivated men and women.

It is likely that in the future legal pressures will require more rigid standard criteria and testing of manual dexterity and competence may help to avoid wastage or the training of the surgically incompetent theorist. It may also be that public pressure will eventually demand psychological profiling, not so much to improve positive selection but to exclude those with character defects and psychopathic personalities.

It is important that selection is to some extent at least seen in a European context. Whatever selection criteria are accepted, they can only be of use if combined with an agreed control of the number of new neurosurgical trainees on a European basis. While the criteria must reflect the cultural differences of the individual countries concerned, they must be strict enough and sufficiently standardised to ensure the same high standard of neurosurgical training continues in all countries. They must be fair and seen to be fair by all eligible candidates and based on merit, competence and ability.

Finally, we should never forget that when candidates whom we would consider as excellent trainees decide against neurosurgery as a career, the fault may lie with us and the perception of our specialty among undergraduates and potential trainees rather than any deficiencies in the candidates themselves.

Correspondence: Dr. T. A. H. Hide, Southern General Hospital, 1345 Govan Road, G51 4TF Glasgow, United Kingdom

Acta Neurochir (1997) [Suppl] 69:8–11

Leadership Qualities in Prominent Neurosurgeons

M. Brock

Department of Neurosurgery, University Hospital Benjamin Franklin, Free University of Berlin, Federal Republic of Germany

Keywords: Leadership Qualities, Prominent Neurosurgeons, Success.

Introduction

The most successful professionals, irrespective of their field of activity, share a set of basic qualities: perfectionism, self-denial and overwork. All are highly competitive, achievement-oriented, easily frustrated, impatient, and suffer from permanent pressure to meet deadlines. These are statements made in a superb paper by J. Maroon, entitled "The Paradox of Success and the Neurosurgeon" [5].

Surprisingly enough, it is difficult to find literature on the topic of leadership and the selection of leaders in medicine. Gabath [3], a psychiatrist who interviewed a large number of successful physicians, concludes that the most successful individuals are determined by society's acceptance, approval, appreciation and applause. This is the case irrespective of their field of activity. As a rule, successful individuals have experienced marked deprivation during childhood.

Deprivation of what?

In most cases, it was deprivation of approval or acceptance regardless of performance. In the formative years, the message was not "I love you because you are you". Rather, the real or perceived message was that approval was achieved only if one lived up to the expectations of parents, teachers, and, subsequently, society at large. In other words, successful leaders strive to meet the expectations of others.

Leadership

Leadership is related to the ability to cooperate, to solve problems, make decisions, integrate, and communicate (Table 1). These are the essentials of leadership, and they are complemented by the personal characteristics of team spirit, flexibility, mobility, responsibility and competence (Table 2).

The above-mentioned characteristics are not developed to the same extent in all leaders. However, none of them is really "underdeveloped" in the presence of real leadership. These aspects have thoroughly been discussed by Böning [2].

Obviously additional qualities such as *engagement*, *creativity*, *perseverance*, and *initiative* are necessary.

Each of the above-mentioned characteristics is, in itself, the complex result of a series of personal abilities. For example, the *ability to solve problems* de-

Table 1. *Prerequisites of Leadership*

Ability to:
– Cooperate
– Solve problems
– Take decisions
– Integrate
– Communicate

Table 2. *Prerequisites of Leadership*

Personal characteristics:
– Team spirit
– Flexibility
– Mobility
– Responsibility
– Competence

pends on creativity, analytical thinking, flexibility, and innovation (Table 3). Also, "competence" (Table 2) not only means profound knowledge or dexterity but includes the concept of *social competence*. This is based on the ability to cooperate, to integrate, to work in a team, and to communicate. Social competence also includes *mobility*. Mobility does not merely signify the physical ability to displace oneself but also the knowledge of foreign languages. Thus, *social competence* and *mobility* are additional prerequisites for a "modern times leader".

Levinson [4] adds *integrity*, *social responsibility*, *perception for achievement*, and *corporate interest*. These are, of course, especially necessary when it comes to leadership of larger groups or enterprises.

According to Benis and Nanus [1], leading personalities adopt certain *main strategies* (Table 4). Obviously, attracting attention of co-workers by means of a visionary goal is paramount in promoting progress, achieving motivation, and creating team spirit. However, a vision, no matter how strong, must be adequately conveyed and is thus useless without communication.

It is generally agreed that nowadays the more "traditional" forms of leadership, in which authority and rationality played a major role, have been replaced by leadership concepts in which emotionality gains importance (Fig. 1). The "cool" leader has lost appeal in the same measure as information has become widely available to almost everybody through modern media.

An attempt was made to interview and compare some of the leading and very successful neurosurgeons, whether they share same common characteristics and whether they could have been recognized already at a very early stage in their lives.

Table 3. *Ability to Solve Problems*

– Creativity
– Analytical thinking
– Flexibility
– Innovation

Table 4. *Main Strategies of Leading Personalities* [1]

1. Attract attention with a vision
2. Convey sense through communication
3. Fill a position and elicit trust
4. Development of the own personality

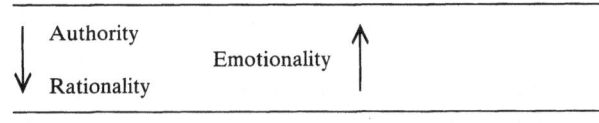

Fig. 1

Material and Methods

A questionnaire containing 10 questions was mailed to 10 neurosurgeons well known to the neurosurgical community worldwide. The 10 questions were:

Questions

1. School life: How was your performance at school? Were you the first in your class? What disciplines were your strength? What were your ratings: first third? second third? third third of your class?
2. What were your ratings in medical school: first third? second third? third third of your class?
3. Sports: Did you actively engage in sports? What discipline? Did you participate in tournaments? Did you win prizes?
4. Hobbies: What were your hobbies in your youth? Are they still your hobbies? Have they influenced your professional activities?
5. Music and literature: Have you learned to play a musical instrument? Have you given concerts? Do you still play? Are you also interested in literature? What is your favorite book? Who is your favorite poet?
6. Others: Are there any other factors that have influenced your career? Are there any "impacts" you have been exposed to during your youth which you consider "decisive" for your success? Are you ambitious?
7. Let me know about the influence your teachers at school had on your medical career and on your success.
8. Please also inform me about the imprints of teachers at medical school on your success and on your decision to become a neurosurgeon.
9. Considering that you are one of the most successful neurosurgeons of our times, what is your "recipe" for success in neurosurgery, and what are the "basic qualities" you consider necessary to become a successful neurosurgeon. Please give a list of the "five basic qualities" a neurosurgeon should possess.
10. Did you notice any "early signs" of your manual skill?

Results

Of the 10 neurosurgeons included in this inquiry, 6 answered all 10 questions. In addition, one discontinued answering the questionnaire between questions 6 and 7 because he had to leave for a congress!

School Life

All neurosurgeons who returned the questionnaire were good or very good at school, sometimes despite material difficulties. The preferred disciplines were the natural sciences. Thus, the school years of these outstanding neurosurgeons were already marked by a fair degree of excellence combined with an interest in biological phenomena.

Medical School

All but one belonged to the upper third in medical school. One disliked lectures and preferred to go to hospitals, where he could establish closer contact with patients. One ran into serious material problems during the 4th year of medical school, since one of his girlfriends had become pregnant. Nevertheless, he has become an outstanding neurosurgeon due largely to strong support from one of his teachers (also an outstanding leader of world-wide renown).

Sports

All interviewed neurosurgeons practiced sports. Two had participated in tournaments, and another won several prizes. They all stress a high level of motivation and orientation towards success.

Hobbies

The following hobbies were mentioned: horseback riding, music (twice), model construction (three times), amateur radio, stamp collecting, walking and golfing. Those who had model construction as their hobby clearly stated that, already during childhood, they had found out that they were manually skilled.

Music and Literature

All were interested in music. Three played a musical instrument well. Four stated they only played the gramophone. All were interested in classical literature, mainly in Shakespeare. In this context, it is interesting to notice that all leading neurosurgeons were interested in the fine arts, and none mentioned pop music.

Ambition

"No one who is determined to be a neurosurgeon can be other than ambitious". This sentence is the answer of one of the interviewed leaders. Another one wrote: "Yes, yes, yes". All admitted to being ambitious.

Influence of School Teachers and University Teachers

All leading neurosurgeons had one or more "decisive" teachers responsible for the professional career they chose. Some wrote very extensively about these "decisive" teachers. Not all those personalities were surgeons themselves. There were at least two neurosurgeons deeply influenced by chairmen of departments of internal medicine.

This shows that leading personalities have been exposed to other leading personalities. The question remains whether this exposure is a matter of coincidence (of fortune?), or whether future leading personalities have an aptitude for identifying and becoming attached to other leading personalities already during their early development.

The "Recipe"

According to all leading neurosurgeons who filled out the questionnaire, the recipe for success is: hard work. "Dedication, dedication, dedication", as stated in one of the answers. In addition, other qualities such as humanitarian interest, loyalty, sense of humor and innovative thinking were considered essential for success. Amazingly enough, none mentioned "good fortune" or "luck" as one of the factors leading to success. This shows a high degree of self-reliance and reveals that these leaders are not prone to leaving anything to chance.

Manual Skill

As already stated when dealing with hobbies, practically all interviewed neurosurgeons noticed early in life that they were manually skilled. One found piano playing to be indicative of it. Another stated: "I was early aware from model-making that manual dexterity was never going to be my problem. I have been a mechanic and a repairman since my early childhood".

Success

"Success is ephemeral, and it might be interesting to predict the number of your chosen 10 who will be remembered in 50 years from now". This sentence, written by one of the interviewed leaders, reveals the dilemma: How much of what one does is of importance for future generations? How much is done for personal satisfaction under the alibi of being useful to others? This dilemma reflects that most, if not all, "leading personalities" remain vulnerable to deprivation despite success. Deprivation of applause, deprivation of approval. Each and every one of these "giants" has an Achilles' heel.

Honesty and Self-Criticism

"In the game of surgery, you must be so honest that it hurts". This was the answer of one of the leading neurosurgeons. In fact, honesty was the common denominator of the answers given to all questionnaires. Honesty toward oneself and toward others appears to be one of the chief traits of all leaders. This confirms the generally accepted view that leaders are *genuine*.

Summary and Conclusions

Our questionnaire provided a unique occasion to unravel the characteristics of leading neurosurgeons. As is also the case for successful leaders in other fields, neurosurgical leaders are good at school, used to being confronted with dilemmas, truthloving, ambitious, and, of course, gifted. They constitute a hard-working elite. The key to success is awareness. Awareness of oneself, awareness of one's surroundings, awareness of the message to be delivered, awareness of the difficulties to be overcome and of their solutions.

Awareness requires mental readiness, and this is directly linked to performance excellence in surgery [6].

References

1. Bennis W, Nanus B (1985) Leaders. New York (cit. [2])
2. Böning U (1993) Exzellent Führen. R. Haufe, Freiburg i.Br., 478 pp
3. Gabbard L. In: Skelly FJ (1993) Mapping medicine's mind field: Dr. Gabbard explores physicians' psychological vulnerabilities. AMA News, October 11:11–15 (cit. [5])
4. Levinson H (1981) Qualifikationskriterien für Topmanager. Harvard Manager 2 (cit. [2])
5. Maroon JC (1994) The paradox of success ... and the neurosurgeon. Perspect Neurol Surg 5:151–162
6. Mc Donald J, Orlick T, Letts M (1995) Mental readiness in surgeons and its links to performance excellence in surgery. J Pediat Orthop 15:691–697

Correspondence: Prof.Dr.med.Dr.h.c. M. Brock, Neurochirurgische Klinik, Universitätsklinikum Benjamin Franklin, Hindenburgdamm 30, D-12200 Berlin, Federal Republic of Germany

Acta Neurochir (1997) [Suppl] 69:12–18
© Springer-Verlag 1997

Criteria to Find Qualified Candidates – Professional Personnel Recruitment Methods Adapted to Neurosurgery

J. M. Gilsbach and **A. Pillong**

Neurosurgical Department, University of Technology, Aachen Federal Republic of Germany

Summary

A neurosurgeon has not received any special training in personnel recruitment at the time he becomes chief of a department. Consequently, a suboptimal personnel policy is most probable. Due to the rapid changes in social behaviour and style of leadership in postwar Europe, he might be ill advised to follow only the example of his successful predecessors, apart from the fact, that this would only be possible if the personalities (of the former and new chief) were similar. To save time and energy for optimal patient care, personnel recruitment can be improved and made more reproducible and reliable by adopting modern, professional non-medical principles. A typical stepwise process of personnel recruitment includes an analysis of the position and function, the definition of demands and offers, the choice of advertising and searching methods, the analysis of the application documents, the interview with the candidate including its re-evaluation and the ongoing evaluation process during the training.

This election process is not only conducted by the chief of a department, but also by senior staff-members and even young, competing assistants. It aims to find the candidate who fits best in the requirements, who will be trained and educated with the least effort and who has the best potential to succeed in the long run.

The only factors seemingly predicting a good development of a candidate are personality, energy (potential, motivation) and intelligence. Therefore, the search should especially aim to discover these – admittedly difficult to detect – qualities.

Keywords: Personnel recruitment, success indicators, personality, energy, intelligence.

Introductory Remarks

Before elaborating criteria to find qualified candidates, we should define what "qualified" means in order to know what we deal with. In our opinion, a qualified candidate is a young assistant who has the potential to become an excellent neurosurgeon, eventually able to run a department successfully.

In retrospect, a successful chairman was therefore most probably a qualified candidate at the beginning of his training. Consequently it would be worth to define qualification criteria on the basis of a number of successful neurosurgical careers. Under this aspect, it would be interesting to retrospectively receive information from their former chiefs why they considered these candidates promising and which selection criteria they used.

This procedure, however, is only sensible if success is a clearly defined quality. But what is success in the neurosurgical field? Is it individual satisfaction, celebrity, acceptance or respect paid by colleagues and/ or non-neurosurgical people, a large number of successful pupils or thousands of well-treated patients – or all together? If already the definition of success is a problem in neurosurgery, it must be even more difficult to look for and to define criteria for a qualified candidate who becomes eventually successful. Vice versa, qualified but potentially unsuccessful candidates probably also do exist. It would be important to know some more or less specific predictors by which such potentially unsuccessful candidates in the future can be prevented from being engaged.

A simple and general formula to define and consequently to find qualified candidates does not exist. A retrospective and admittedly subjective analysis of the everyday practice of personnel recruitment the senior author (JMG) has experienced reveals that no specific set of rules can be deduced. Rules, principles and instructions as engagement criteria comparable to those in the industrial, military or show business do not exist in the neurosurgical field. This was the reason to contact the co-author, the chief of a personnel management company to co-operate with neurosurgeons in the field of personnel recruitment. The following is a synthesis of professional recruit-

Table 1. *Stepwise Process of Recruiting Qualified Candidates*

I	analysis of position & function. Profile of demands & offers
II	analysis of existing methods including their results
III	market analysis search strategy
IV	interpretation of application documents, biography, exams information, references, inquiries telephone/written interview, questionnaire personal interview, assessment center tests, proof of skills
V	evaluation during qualifying/training period assessment of ongoing education & training process

Table 2. *Demands and Qualification of a Suited Candidate*

formal	sex, marital status, age, nationality, health
personal	intellect: intelligent, structured, analytic, systematic, discerning, decisive, creative, imaginative, interested, solid general education energy, motivation: engaged, goal-directed, purposeful, stress-resistant, tenacious, patient personality: friendly, convincing, loyal, sincere, authentic, thoughtful, critical, non-professional fields of interest social competence: communicative, able to work in a team, able to lead & motivate, ready to help, emphatic, professional attitude
professional	completed doctoral dissertation, good exam, skill, manual dexterity, capacity of spatial cognition, publications, good English proficiency, stays abroad, PC experience

ment methods combined with special neurosurgical requirements. It is an attempt with recommendations which are – strictly spoken – not scientifically proven.

Proposed Methods to find Qualified Candidates

The search for a qualified candidate does not begin with his introduction. In principle, we must first elaborate strategies of how to address suitable candidates and, second, methods to filter out of this group the most qualified candidate, fulfilling all our requirements. This needs a clear definition of what we want and offer, an analysis of exemplary and effective methods (e.g. of our predecessors or marketing specialists and one's own experience, an analysis of the market situation, a definition of search strategies), the selection process itself and the ongoing evaluation during the training process (Table 1).

a) Expectations of and Offers to the Candidate

Expectations, demands and offers of the recruiting department should be defined before the search for a candidate is initiated. Clearly defined requirements are important prerequisites for a reproducible and focused selection and assessment process. Without rules and standards for both the assistant and the chairman any judgement is arbitrary. In order to attract talented applicants, it is also necessary to present a clear perspective in terms of career and training.

The definition of requirements implies that we know which position and function should be replaced or newly installed. It is obvious that a candidate often does not necessarily fit into all categories. Therefore, the selection criteria depend on the function the candidate should fulfil. Are we looking for a resident eventually entering private practice, for a brilliant

research oriented fellow, a promising assistant professor or a potential academic chairman?

The definition of requirements is also necessary to make clear what is expected from the candidate. In the case of undefined tasks, both the assistant and the faculty will permanently be disappointed. Among the demands, knowledge and experience are less important than personality, intelligence, energy and motivation. Knowledge can be acquired and increased, but not personality and inborn gifts. This becomes especially obvious in leading positions. The higher a neurosurgeon climbs up the career ladder, the more important becomes his personal style. The negative example is the colleague, who is only professionally competent.

A well organised training and promotion for a potential career are things which can be offered by the recruiting department. This is the compensation for long-lasting hard work and possible frustrations the resident has to bear.

This article is aimed to describe criteria for the search of candidates for leading positions, necessarily encompassing all qualities of a good neurosurgeon and the potential of a prospective chief (Table 2)

b) Searching Methods of the Predecessors

Despite existing modern personnel recruitment and development methods, it is worth to evaluate retrospectively chiefs and departments with a high proportion of successful residents. The question is, whether they followed – consciously or unconsciously – rules worth to be adopted.

During his neurosurgical training, the senior author (JMG) experienced two chiefs. Both eventually had many, very successful pupils in terms of getting leading positions and both belonged to the group of leading German neurosurgeons. Therefore it seemed to be worth to analyse exemplarily their methods.

– The Gießen Experience:

The first chief was a general-like type, who personally hired his assistants after a 20-minute interview. During this time he evaluated mainly the sociodemographic background of the candidate. Almost no engaged candidate was fired later on. It is neither known how many applicants were not accepted nor what the criteria were to preselect them. Eventually, seven of his former pupils became chairmen in university hospitals and two became chiefs in community hospitals. Five of the nine successful pupils stayed in this institution when they received their final position.

The secret of success of the Gießen chairman was to hire – but not to fire –, to press and promote his assistants. In retrospect, I can, however, not prove whether preselection or pressing was the main element of his success. As a drawback, this system had an inherent risk of promoting untalented neurosurgeons.

– The Freiburg Experience:

The second chief favoured a mixture of co-operative and laissez-faire style in running his department. Correspondingly, he hired or let the senior staff members hire new assistants and observed their progress. The selection of the candidates was roughly done on the basis of exam results and certificates after a short talk. On account of the small number of applicants, most of the candidates were engaged according to the motto: trial and error.

Within two years it became obvious whether or not the young assistants were able to fulfil their tasks. Then, a preliminary, not organised assessment was made, mostly by senior assistants and assistant professors. On the basis of this information, most of the assistants were advised to leave the institution. This could also happen after the assistant had completed his training and passed the board examination. Altogether 90% of the beginners did not succeed to stay on in Freiburg, before they moved to their definitive position.

Within 15 years, four of the neurosurgeons who started their training in Freiburg became chairmen in university hospitals and six in community hospitals, respectively. Interestingly, only two of those ten successful beginners obtained their leading position directly from Freiburg University. The other eight first had moved to other departments to continue a career whose foundation, however, was laid in Freiburg. The secret of success of the Freiburg chairman was to hire, to observe and to correct engagement errors by firing or pressing away. Despite the lack of clearly defined selection criteria, the Freiburg system was extremely effective in terms of eventually producing chiefs. Instead of a sophisticated selection process, the trial and error principle was used. The assistant was hired, put under working pressure, was intensively observed and if considered necessary stimulated to leave after 2 to 5 years. This system, however, turned out to be extremely "costly" because of a permanent fluctuation among the residents and the staff. Although successful and effective, this method was not efficient, neither for the

teacher nor the pupil nor the patient. Hundreds of hours were wasted by training, correcting and controlling those unsuccessful assistants. Beside the time loss, psychological stress arose from the fear of a reduced treatment quality. This Freiburg experience proves once more that efficacy is not necessarily associated with efficiency.

The assistants and co-workers of my former chiefs made a successful career either by election, selection or designation by their chief in the teaching hospital. It seems that their methods to find and promote qualified candidates were more or less emotional or instinctive, but not rational and reproducible. Their methods were effective in terms of career, but not necessarily in terms of personality development, effort and patient care. In the first institution, there was an inherent risk to press the wrong neurosurgeon to a career, because a potentially unwise selection was not corrected by firing. In the second institution, the effort did not equal the effect, because often time and energy were invested in the education of an untalented assistant.

In review, the senior author was and still is not able to predict the career of the individual beginner. After 25 professional years, at least 50% of the initial judgement was wrong in retrospect. The only factors seemingly predictive of a good development of a candidate are energy (potential, motivation) and intelligence.

These two personal experiences represent typical examples of personnel policy in the late sixties, seventies and early eighties in Germany. Today, a chief is aware that by obtaining a leading position, he is not necessarily endowed with inborn qualities as a headhunter for promising candidates. On the other side, there is a definite need to select the right candidate from the beginning, in order not to lose undue energy. The question is, can we adapt modern selection techniques or do we need professional help?

c) Influence of Personal Experiences on Personnel Recruitment Methods

A major share of our professional and private behaviour and judgement is influenced by our parents, teachers, role models etc. We often follow and copy unconsciously what we have seen, heard and experienced. Therefore, it is important to analyse critically our own personal background to better understand the rules we follow unnoticed and the mistakes we make traditionally. This may be helpful to avoid repetition of traditional faults and may lead to a realistic view. We may, for instance, ask how successful we have been with our selection process. The capability to select qualified candidates can be determined by the ratio of successful pupils in leading academic positions divided by the number of engaged residents. The ideal quotient would be 1:1. A ratio of 1:10 probably is more realistic. Such a retrospective analysis of the development of previous co-workers is useful to calibrate one's own capability to select talented candidates.

d) Professional Attempts to find Qualified Candidates

In contrast to the past, where the selection process was based mainly on intuition and experience, modern personnel recruitment strategies rely more on clearly defined criteria and demands. However, such criteria have to be defined for our particular purpose. These selection criteria should be based – if possible – on predictors of positive and successful development.

The selection process begins with the definition of the situation, position and demands in the searching department and includes announcements and advertisements. It is followed by an analysis of the documents of the candidates and it is completed by interviews and probably also by tests. Logically, it should be supplemented by a certain observation period of the least 6 months.

e) Where and how do we look for a good Candidate?

For a musical, up to 300 people are evaluated in order to cast a top role. For an equally important neurosurgical position, often less than 1/10 candidates apply if no specific search strategy is followed. So, the first step of a successful search must be to increase the number of potentially qualified applicants (Table 3).

– The wrong search at the right time or vice versa are severe hindrances to a successful engagement.

Table 3. *Search Strategy*

market analysis	right time, potential candidates available, geographical region attractive?
search method	chance, purpose, advertising, announcing, enticing, head hunting

Therefore, either repeated announcements or targeted advertisements are necessary.
– From the few announcements in relevant journals, it may be assumed that usually the qualified candidate is chosen from spontaneously emerging applicants. This is to some extent a selection by chance with a reduced prospect to find the best candidate for a specific position.
– The announcement should contain a realistic description of the position and its requirements. This probably decreases the number of unqualified candidates and increases the pool from which qualified candidates can be chosen.
– The department itself or its environment (city, culture etc.) may be attractive enough to induce a qualified candidate from another department to apply. This method has the advantage that the candidate already has been observed in his performance. It bears, however, the risk of creating frictions.

f) How can we evaluate the Individual Candidate?

The next step is the evaluation of the individual candidate. In principle, it consists of four phases:

1. analysis & interpretation of documents
2. interview
3. short stay, test, probationary work
4. ongoing evaluation & assessment

– The interpretation of examination results and the curriculum vitae is a very important part. The documents not only inform on the course of the professional life of the candidate but also unfold to a certain extent his personality (Table 4).
– A good interview needs a preparation period without the candidate, a contact, information and closing period with the candidate and a re-evaluation process of the complete interview without the candidate but with all interviewers (Table 5).

Table 4. *Analysis of Documents*

- outer appearance, formal order, completeness
- covering letter
- curriculum vitae, continuous employment
- professional and personal prerequisites
- exam results, reports, certificates, references
- personnel questionnaire
- handwriting
- photo

Table 5. *Elements of an Interview*

I	preparation period
II	contact period, information period, closing period
III	retrospective analysis

Table 6. *Preparation of the Interview*

- invitation of more than one candidate?
- invitation with spouses?
- provision of time & undisturbed, friendly atmosphere
- evaluation of documents, references
- predetermined topics, agenda
- delegation of tasks
- standardised (open) questions
- paper & pencil for notes
- aim at a positive image of the own department!

Table 7. *Topics of an Interview*

- biographical data
- social background
- special activities, hobbies
- foreign languages
- description of the position/function
- expectations
- professional qualification
- motivation
- dates
- decision?

Table 8. *Advices for the Interviewer*

- be direct & lead the interview by questions
- prefer open questions
- don't ask rhetoric questions
- avoid monologues
- make notes
- learn active listening and being silent
- observe body language, face
- also address delicate topics
- avoid personal judgements/statements

Table 9. *Evaluation of an Interview*

person,	punctuality, outer appearance,
personality	behaviour, body language, authenticity,
	leadership qualities, energy, motivation
intellect	intelligence, structured mind
specialist	experience, surgical talent
potential,	power, charisma, health, persistency
prospects	innovative & creative qualities
qualification	as specialist & person?

data. In this respect (for a better comparability), it can be an advantage to interview consecutively up to 4 candidates. The interviewer should be familiar with the curriculum vitae. It is a key to the personality of the candidate and can be used to specifically address interesting aspects. At least two people should lead the interview (Table 6).

- The interview with the candidate himself consists of three parts: the contact period, the information period and the closing period. During the contact period, the applicant is informed about the subsequent steps, is introduced to other participants, etc. Also, first impressions are registered, e.g. facial expression and strength of handshake. The *information process* follows a clear order which helps to improve the gathering of facts and their interpretation. It is directed by means of open questions and begins with biographical and sociodemographic data and formal aspects of the professional career (Table 7).
- An interview should principally be directed and led by open questions. The candidate and not the interviewer must have the chance to present himself. Three quarters of the time have to be reserved for the candidate. Personal comments and statements of the interviewer are not helpful to evaluate the candidate (Table 8).
- During the closing period of an interview the interviewer expresses his thanks to the candidate and informs him when a decision will be reached. Normally, definite acceptance of the candidate is not expressed at the end of the interview.
- The result of the analysis of documents, information and the interview should immediately be summarised and re-evaluated at the end of the interview after a discussion with the other participants. The question has to be answered whether the candidate fulfils the criteria for engagement. A later and final conference should compare all ac-

- The interview is one of the most important milestones of the search for qualified candidates. It should be thoroughly prepared and be concentrated on the candidate. A friendly and undisturbed atmosphere is a prerequisite for a meaningful interview. Standardised topics and open questions are useful to obtain comparable

ceptable candidates and end up with a ranking list including all pros and cons (Table 9).

– Personality is a given dimension and an extremely important factor. Many of the unsuccessful pupils rather fail because of their character than lack of skill and knowledge. As chiefs, we tend to believe too much in our teaching and educating qualities and consequently are too optimistic to find the brilliant candidate among applicants with average exam results and a standard uneventful curriculum vitae. We should trust less in our training program and emphasize more the pre-selection and selection process. Typical mistakes in decision making and advices to prevent them are shown in Table 10 and 11.

– At the end of the selection process, the candidate-elect should also be frankly informed about the situation during the 6-year training period: it must be made clear that he is expected to work hard, to tolerate and suffer a lot, that he must be tough and tenacious and train his mind and skill and that all this may happen on the expense of family life and, perhaps, will influence to some extent the development of his personality.

– More advanced candidates for higher positions can better be investigated in terms of professional qualities. If possible, a visit to the former department with observation of the candidate in his familiar working atmosphere, interviews with his colleagues and nurses are helpful to evaluate the qualities of the applicant.

Conclusions

Well defined criteria and methods are very important to increase the proportion of successful residents. They help to reduce inefficient efforts to train and educate untalented persons. They help also to prevent patients from being harmed by ungifted surgeons.

They are, however, only prerequisites for a successful career of a good neurosurgeon. Only a neurosurgical department with a high clinical and training standard transforms a gifted assistant into a good neurosurgeon (Table 12, 13). Otherwise, even a very talented young assistant has no chance to become a competent academic neurosurgeon. Therefore, candidates are well advised to invest energy and time to find a qualified department with a good training programme.

Table 10. *Typical Mistakes During an Interview*

- try to find your character and characteristics in the candidate
- believe too much in your educating and teaching qualities
- forget, that character and personality are given factors
- underestimate the importance of social competence
- invest in unsuited candidates, they will not reward

Table 11. *Advices to Prevent Typical Mistakes During an Interview*

- invite young assistants (competitors) to check the candidate
- invite senior colleagues to take part in the interview
- accept that the candidate presents himself
- react, don't speak to much
- find out the potential, the developmental reserves
- believe more in inborn qualities and less in development

Table 12. *Principles to Find Qualified Candidates*

D	define	what we are looking for, what and who is needed
E	evaluate	market situation, documents, references, information
S	speak	with the candidate
I	inform	the candidate about his rights and duties
R	relegate	candidates who are wrongly chosen
E	encourage	promising candidates

Table 13. *Steps to have Qualified Candidates, Making a Successful Career*

S	select	a healthy, intelligent, tenacious, dynamic, psychologically intact and sincere candidate, with manual dexterity, resistant to psychological and physical stress
T	teach	him structured, critical and scientific thinking
E	educate	him as a good doctor and neurosurgeon
P	promote	him

It has to be stressed that the above described psychologically based, businesslike recruitment methods are not yet validated to find gifted neurosurgical assistants. Time will tell us whether these modern selection methods are superior to the intuitive classical method. On the basis of his experience and observations, the senior author (JMG) comes to the conclusion that it is the combination of intelligence with motivation and manual dexterity which characterises best the qualified candidate.

Correspondence: Prof. J. M. Gilsbach, Neurosurgical Department, University Hospital, University of Technology (RWTH) Aachen, Pauwelsstrasse 30, D-52057 Aachen, Federal Republic of Germany

Acta Neurochir (1997) [Suppl] 69:19–21

Criteria and Procedures in the Automotive Industry

I. Kohlhofer

BMW AG, München, Federal Republic of Germany

Keywords: Selection process, automotive industry, performance criteria.

The purpose of this contribution is to give a short impression on how BMW AG selects and develops upcoming executives. For our company this is essential for the future, it is therefore of strategic significance.

The only way to establish and maintain an edge in competition in the long run is through careful selection and continuous development of all employees' skills. What BMW needs, quite simply, is the right executive at the right place and at the right time. We need executives with a strong personality, executives who give an example. Unfortunately, such executives are not just born as they are, they do not suddenly appear out of the dark.

One challenge within this process is *selection*, the other one is *continuous development*.

BMW is convinced that we have to handle both challenges. They are like two sides of the same coin.

Table 1 shows the performance criteria for executives. They provide a common, uniform basis for all selection and development processes (within management). They can be tailored to each individual selection process by considering specific demands und ranking.

What BMW needs are employees who are capable of entrepreneurial thinking and acting, who have an overall process – and technical competence and additionally – which is very important-who are showing constructive leadership and team behaviour.

We are assessing *performance* at one hand and the *impact of personality* on the other hand. We are strongly convinced that success – or let me put it this way – *effectiveness* is based on both criteria.

The responsibility for selection and development processes is with different executives and personnel departments because BMW is a decentralised organisation. Therefore we need principles in terms of guidelines (Table 2).

We are lucky to have lots of applications. Most of them are of a high quality. So, how to find the right candidate?

The first guideline is the most important one: *personality is essential, specialism is a basic requirement.*

It is not enough to do the right thing, it is also important to do it in the right way and to do it together with different partners who are working for the same target but often from a quite different point of view.

The first step within the selection process is the definition of the demand criteria. The profile of the future candidate must be agreed upon by *all the people involved* in the process. Otherwise it is not possible to gain acceptance.

We are looking for different candidates – those with a broader spectrum and those who are able to work in specific jobs within a process chain (i.e. production – from central planning to assembly line).

The selection teams are always mixed in order to assess the candidates under different points of view.

For selection BMW uses mainly three methods – assessment center (group and single) and situational interviews. These methods are more cost- and work intensive. We at BMW are convinced that for specific groups of candidates these methods justify the higher investment. Because they are more reliable in the prediction of the professional potential and professional success. And we achieve also a higher objectiv-

Table 1. *Demand/Performance Criteria for Executives*

Entrepreneurial thinking and acting	Target achievement results (qualitative/quantitative) Process/technical competence	Leadership and team behaviour
For example: > Overall company-related thinking and action Ability to develop a vision > Taking the customer as a yardstick > Process management, management of change > Cost and result awareness	For example: > Process know-how > Process oriented approach > Zero-mistake attitude > Ability to analyse and take decisions, assessment and acceptance of risks	For example: > Target agreements > Dialogue and team ability > Employee motivation, development

Impact of personality			
credible	consistent	open/assessable	integration – oriented

Table 2. *Principles and Guidelines*

personality is essential
specialism is a basic requirement
clear definition of the demand criteria
mixed selection teams (holistic view)
selection team consists of executives
from related departments (process chain)

ism and avoid therefore the so-called "gut-decisions". Gut – decisions are sometimes very helpful, but it strongly depends on whose gut is making the decision.

To sum it up, the challenge in terms of selection is to achieve high process quality and objectivity. But as mentioned before, selection is only the beginning. Without continuous personnel development selection is nearly a dead end street. At BMW we have established what we call a discussion round process (Table 3). The process consists of five steps starting in September each year and concluded by year end. The targets of these rounds are to get an *overall view* in terms of *performance* (qualitative and quantitative target achievement results) and *future potential*.

Table 3. *Discussion Round Process*

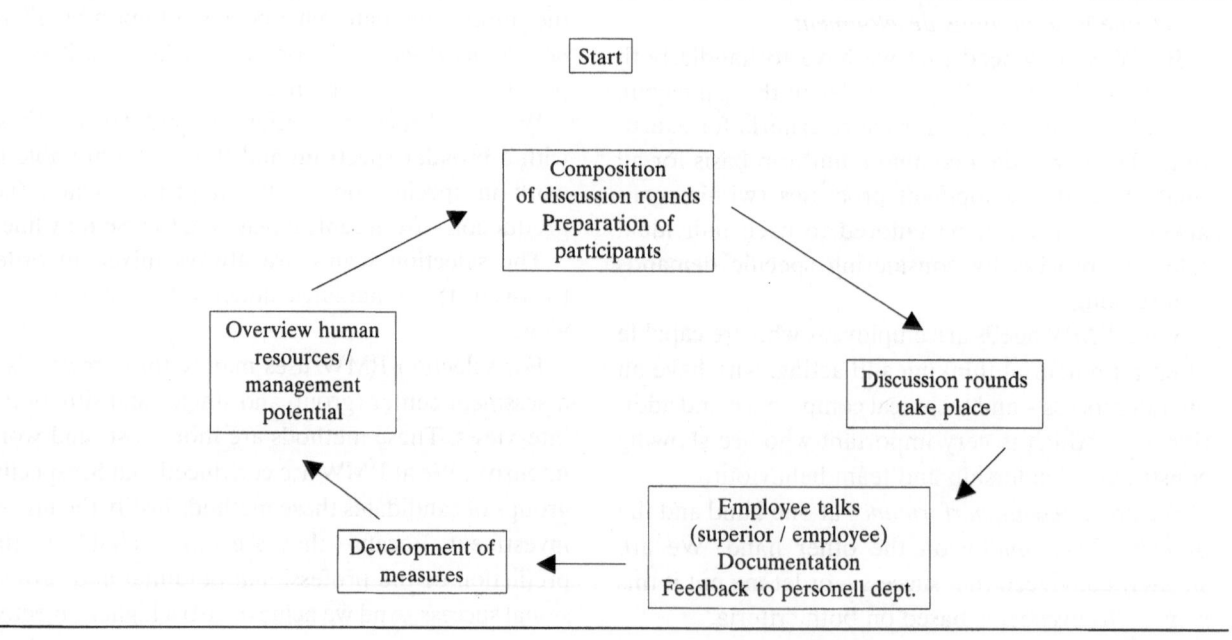

Since all managers regardless of hierarchy level both in Germany and abroad are measured by the same criteria and standards, we obtain a clear-cut picture of the entire company, messages and information of enhanced quality and as results:

- more possibilities for developing management potentials beyond the limits of divisions or specific processes and

- we get more qualified information if our selection processes are working.

Correspondence: I. Kohlhofer, c/o BMW AG München, PZ 36 BMW AG München, D-80788 München, Federal Republic of Germany

Acta Neurochir (1997) [Suppl] 69:22–26
© Springer-Verlag 1997

Selection of Air Force Officers – Profiles, Criteria, Testing

H.-W. Jarosch

German Air Force Academy, Fürstenfeldbruck, Federal Republic of Germany

Summary

The article presents an explanation of the selection process for German Air Force (GAF) officers in general, and those for flying duty in particular. The text includes an overview of the entire selection and training process, the desired profiles and characteristics of GAF officers, criteria for evaluating current officers, and statistics which show the results of this process.

Keywords: Officers, profiles, criteria, testing.

There are undoubtedly distinct differences between the factors for determining neurosurgical training candidates and those for air force officers' training and education. Quite a number of the requirements may, however, be similar or allow for analogies. Some could even prove to be identical. Any comparison and conclusions are left to one's own judgment.

Selection and training of personnel is a key to successful operations in any organization. The quality desired for the final product determines the quality of the selection process. The more complex and important the duties of the individual to be selected are, the more decisive and difficult the selection and training process must be. If one succeeded in selecting only candidates who completely comply with *every* requirement of their later tasks, one would not only reach optimum professional performance, but could equally minimize losses during the training process. These criteria reflect the proposals of F. Steege ([1], p86) from his current and future selection criteria for military leaders.

In the German Air Force, highest attention is devoted to this subject. The objectives – optimum professional performance and minimized attrition during the training process – are extremely important. The preparation of one single officer for flying duty costs between 1.5 and 2 million DM[1] – and we need approximately 100 new flight crew members per year. Hence, there is a strong need for a reliable selection system.

The following considerations deal exclusively with the selection of air crew members within the German Air Force. It has to be pointed out that out of the approximately 10,000 officers of the Luftwaffe only about 20% are air crew members, and that the other specialties have basically the same problem of selection and training. Flying duty, however, has the most sophisticated requirements and, therefore, the furthest developed selection system.

Before explaining the three aspects of the selection process – definition of profiles, criteria and testing, the testing and training sequence for our future air force officers needs to be explained.

Figure 1 shows the hurdles that each air crew candidate has to overcome before he may begin his operational duty. But even the necessary post-graduate training is rather extensive, as shown on the right hand side of the chart. This advanced part of the training process that ultimately will make the young officer "mission capable" is not part of this paper, although it is very important for the proficiency of the individual and the entire unit.

There are three examinations to pass before entering service. Normally, these tests are taken twelve to six months prior. The first one is a test that every officer candidate has to take at the German Armed Forces Officers Test Center at Cologne. The other two are given only to air crew candidates at the Ger-

---

[1] These figures include costs for basic military training, leadership training, flight screening and flying training

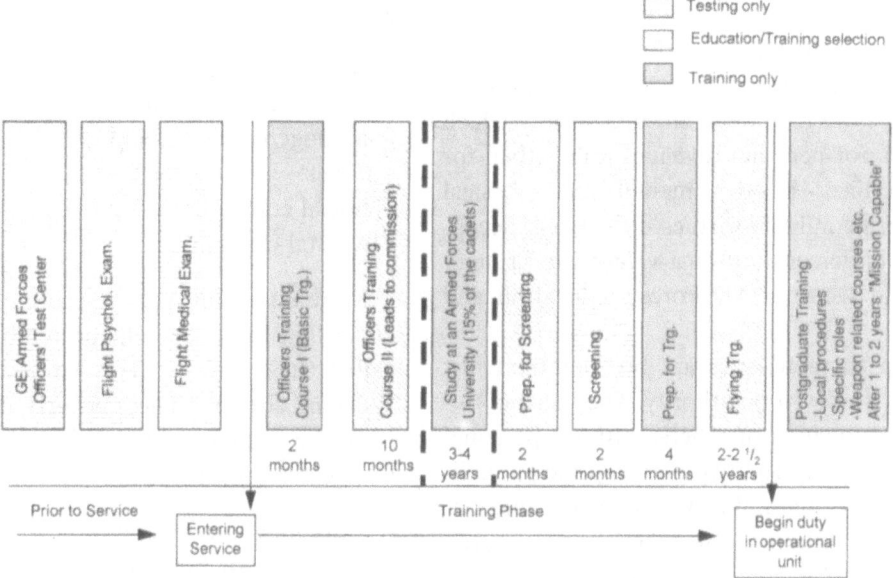

Fig. 1. Selection, testing and training sequence for German Air Force officers

man Air Force Institute of Aviation Medicine at Fürstenfeldbruck. They are the flight psychological examination and the flight medical examination.

After entering the service, the officer candidate, now called a "cadet," starts a training phase that lasts between $4^{1}/_{2}$ and 8 years. The remarkable difference between the extremes in duration is caused by the fact that about 15% of the aviation cadets will attend a degree program at the Armed Forces University. Aside from this period at the university, the sequence is the same for all air crew members. It starts with the officers' basic training, and a 10-month leadership course ending with the comprehensive officers' examination. After this common training period some of the aviation cadets attend the Armed Forces University. The majority remains at the Air Force Academy to start their preparation for screening. Since a good command of the English language is mandatory, some cadets need additional language training. Within the preparation for screening, and in addition to the academic instruction, there is a preselection process with a *flight psychological simulator*, the FPS 80. The screening itself is conducted in the United States at Goodyear, Arizona, and comprises academics and practical flying, normally ending with a student solo flight.

Those who pass the screening return to the Air Force Academy and are prepared for their

flying training, either as a fighter pilot, weapon systems operator, transport or helicopter pilot. Only the transport pilots are trained in Germany at the Lufthansa Pilot School in Bremen. All the others return for their flying training to the United States.

Figure 1 also shows the role that individual events play in the selection process. There are events which are strictly for testing, those that are a mixture of training, education and selection, and others for the pure training phases. After having presented you with the full sequence, let me now emphasize the philosophy behind it, and then expand on those phases that are most important for the selection of German Air Force officers.

Testing of future air crews needs to be based on solid criteria which must be derived from a defined notion of the expected profile of the typical air crew member. The first step, therefore, is to define the profiles.

Each air force officer has to be a military individual, a military leader and a specialist.

To be a military individual means to voluntarily accept the mission of the Air Force, which includes having responsibility for others and acting under possible risk of one's own health or life. As a member of the military in a democratic country, ethical acceptance of the basic values of our constitution is another prerequisite. From the officer candidate not only the readiness for personal sacrifice is expected, but equally the acceptance of the values behind our mission. These are high demands in a society which prefers to ask for personal revenues rather than for personal sacrifice. Besides mental and physical fitness and basic military virtues, the ethical acceptance of the basic constitutional values is a primary subject of the German Air Force's education and training.

Leadership characteristics are broader than just the capability to develop authority. They include responsibility, motivation of others, setting a personal example and resolve. The two parts – principal military requirements and military leadership – are developed in the 12-month officer training, primarily conducted at the Air Force Academy.

For those cadets designated for flying duty there are additional characteristics to consider. They have to comply with special physical requirements and with the flight psychological requirements such as spatial orientation, coordination etc. In addition, they have to be highly resistant to stress.

One must keep in mind, that the selection of future air force officers is based not only on today's requirements, but also on those of our future missions. These officers-to-be will have to take responsibility in an environment where computers double their operating speed every 18 months. Within their service time air forces will be using space-based reconnaissance systems, new information systems, stealthy carriers and intelligent weapons. Technological development will have an enormous impact on military operations across the full spectrum, and in particular on air force operations. Therefore, all the previously mentioned characteristics will become even more important in the future.

From this very brief description of the desired profile of future air force officers were derived two categories of criteria for the selection process:

– basic military criteria and
– specific criteria for flying duty.

The basic military criteria are the ones used for the German Air Force officers' efficiency reports. These criteria cover the characteristics required. This list contains all the keywords mentioned before, and could easily be used to evaluate leaders or management personnel anywhere outside the military.

Basic Criteria:

– Responsibility
– Leadership capability
– Management capabilities
– Trust
– Social competence
– Mental capabilities

More interesting may be the *specific criteria for air crews* that have been elaborated by a NATO forum called the "Euro-NATO Aircrew Human Factors Working Group."[2] These criteria are directly derived from the profile defined for flight crews, and cover their essential capabilities. They include:

– Situational awareness
– Time Sharing (Task management)
– Spatial orientation
– Visualization
– Psychomotor coordination
– Memorization
– Reasoning
– Perceptual speed
– Selective attention
– Responsive orientation.

These criteria hold true for any air crew, civilian or military. The previously mentioned working group therefore has defined additional criteria for air crews beyond aircraft handling.

– Challenge acceptance (aggressiveness)
– Self confidence
– Leadership
– Motivation
– Stress resistance
– Resolve (decisiveness)

These criteria are of special significance for military air crews, and are all certainly vital for a fighter pilot.

The necessity to combine basic military criteria and specific aviation criteria is occasionally questioned. The German Air Force, however, chose this universal approach with the two pillars "leadership characteristics" and "functional competence."

As regards the many events involved in the testing sequence, it would be impossible to present and ana-

---

[2] The Euro-NATO Aircrew Human Factors Working Group was established in 1985 with the aim of evaluating and implementing selection procedures for flying training candidates

lyze all of them in detail within this presentation. Therefore, only three of the different testing phases are discussed below as examples.

The first area is the psychological examination given at the Armed Forces Officers' Test Center, which is just one out of nine different parts[3] that the officer candidate must pass during his stay at the test center. But it is probably the most analytical test, and some of the subjects tested are relevant to basic officership as well as to air crew suitability [2]. The psychological test procedure has a psychometric basis. It is conducted using a computer assisted facility within the test center. This particular test is strictly performance oriented and does not query personal interests or character. The test contains mathematics, logic and comprehension.

All the test areas at the center are periodically evaluated by comparing the results with those reached by the individual at the Officers Academy. This way the selection process is regularly validated. The reliability of these tests is acceptable; and ranges from 0.6 to 0.8.

The second area is the flight psychological test given at the GAF Institute of Aviation Medicine, Flight Psychology Department, in Fürstenfeldbruck. The psychologist who judges the candidate's suitability has the test results from the Test Center available. The candidate must undergo sensory-motor tests as well as conduct simple flight maneuvers in a simulator under instrument flight conditions. Reliability of this test partially stems from a high repetition rate – the candidate has to conduct altogether 32 different "flights" with the system.

There is no final validation of the flight psychological test. One may conclude from the individual results of those who passed the test as compared to their follow-on results within screening and flying training, that the flight psychological test is a fairly reliable tool to coarsely identify the suitability of the candidates for flying duty.

As pointed out in Fig. 1, the *preparation* for screening currently is not an official selection phase. In this two-month preparation phase, however, the flight psychological selection system (FPS-80) has proven to be an excellent indicator for the further

selection steps. The FPS-80 again is a computer assisted psychological test system. It works on a visual mode of control-basis and contains all essential instruments and aircraft handling systems. The candidates undergo academic training which familiarizes them with the basics of aerodynamics and navigation. This academic training includes learning of the FPS-80 flight data (power settings, flight instruments, etc.). This phase concludes with two written tests. The practical phase comprises five different missions that have to be "flown" under supervision of an instructor pilot and a psychologist. Out of the large number of criteria that are applied, there are some particularly relevant, i.e. continuous concentration, time sharing (or task management), movement control, but also self-control and training progress. From the results reached during the following tests and

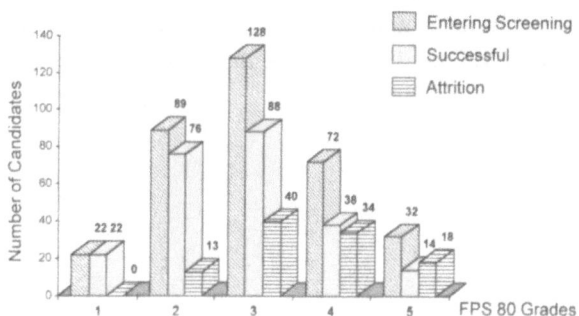

From F.-J. Daumann, W. Greß, B. Willkomm. German Air Force Institute of Aviation Medicine, LEK-Report 1995

Fig. 2. Comparison of FPS-80 grades to flight screening success. From LEK Report 1995 [4]. The grades are awarded 1 through 5, with 1 being the best possible grade and 3 indicating average performance

Complete Selection Process
(per 100 candidates)

	Sequential Steps	Entering Number	Passing
1	GE Armed Forces Officers Test Center	100	20%
2	Flight Psychology	20	70%
3	Flight Medical	14	70%
4	Officer Training	10	85-90%
5	Screening	9	60%
6	Flying Training	5	80% (plus)

Out of 100 candidates for flying duty only about 4-5 will be aircrew members in an operational unit

Fig. 3. Success rate at each step throughout the entire process

---

[3] The other parts of the officer candidate test at the Armed Forces Officer Test Center include an initial medical examination, physical fitness test, evaluation of personal references, producing an essay on a given subject, a round table discussion, group behavior analysis, an interview and a presentation

during flying training, experts have derived a reliability of about 0.9 – an extraordinarily high value. The actual comparison between FPS-80-results and the screening at Goodyear, Arizona, are shown on the chart in Fig. 2. These results currently are driving considerations to exclude those candidates who fail in either phase from the further selection process.

Conclusion

As regards the total results of the selection process, out of 100 applicants for flying duty in the German Air Force only 4 to 5 will ultimately make it all the way to an operational unit (see Fig. 3).

Besides the German Air Force Officers' Test Center which eliminates about 80% of the applicants, the major attrition stems from flight psychology and flight medical tests as well as from the screening. The system has proven its validity. Nevertheless we are continuously analyzing opportunities for improvement. Making better use of the FPS-80 results is one step in this direction. Other nations' selection systems are looked at, for example Schmiedjell [3], and the German Air Force's own system is periodically evaluated.

Success is important – for the selection process of today will determine the quality of the Luftwaffe for the next 30 to 35 years.

References

1. Steege F (1988) Auswahlkriterien für Führungspersonal in den Streitkräften. Innere Führung (Koblenz): 85–123
2. Kriesel W, Lippert E, Klein P (1993) Auslese an der Offizierbewerberprüfzentrale: Offizierbewerber und Offizieranwärter (1992) – Ein empirischer Vergleich. SOWI Arbeitspapier Nr. 79:18–19
3. Schmiedjell A (1996) Personalauswahl – ein Fremdwort? Truppendienst (Wien) 219:223–224
4. Greß W, Willkomm B (1995) Langzeiterfolgskontrolle für den Fliegerischen Dienst (LEK). LEK-Bericht 1995, Flugmedizinisches Institut der Luftwaffe Fürstenfeldbruck, pp 25–28

Correspondence: Brigadegeneral H.-W. Jarosch, Commandant, German Air Force Academy, P.O. Box 1264 A/S, D-82242 Fürstenfeldbruck, Federal Republic of Germany

Acta Neurochir (1997) [Suppl] 69:27–29

Can We Define or Measure Manual Skills in Surgical Training?

G. Neil-Dwyer and **D. A. Lang**

Wessex Neurological Centre, Southampton University Hospitals, Southamptom, United Kingdom

Summary

Neurosurgery requires manual dexterity. But should tests be devised to assess manual skills as part of a selection process for training or used as a means of determining surgical competence?

The paper debates this fundamental question and proposes that manual skills for neurosurgical tasks need to be defined within the overall context of a recognised and fully assessed training programme. The importance of training as a means of transferring competence, part of which is manual skills, is emphasised. In conclusion the paper points out the inadequacy of solely measuring manual skills, were it possible, in assessing neurosurgical competence.

Keywords: Manual skills, skill assessment, manual dexterity.

There has been increasing public, political and medical concern about surgical competence over recent years. The concern is centred on two areas, the perceived wide variation in skill between one surgeon and another and the competence of surgeons to undertake relatively new untried procedures such as minimal invasive surgery. The skill and competence of surgeons are often assumed as being due to special manual skills and there is a view that surgical results are directly related to manual dexterity. While the evidence for this lacks evaluated support, it has led to a concept that manual skills need to be assessed in the selection of surgical trainees.

Manual skills should be regarded as synonymous with dexterity which is defined as being the skill and ease in using the hands or body – technical proficiency and mental adroitness cleverness in dealing with people. The definition highlights the importance and complex relationship between cerebral and manual activity.

How important is dexterity in surgery? Some would argue that we are born with it as a natural gift.

Others contend that it is in all of us to recognise, work on and improve. This leads to a fundamental question. Should the debate on manual skills be centred on a skill assessment for entry into neurosurgical training or should it be directed at the development of the skill in the young trainee surgeon?

Neurosurgeons need a degree of manual dexterity, but is it the case that by and large this occurs by a process of natural selection? This question can to a large extent be answered by examining some of the psycho-motor assessment data that is available.

There is no evidence to suggest that medical students select surgical specialities according to their skills. Dental schools have used skill tests in assessments of candidates entering basic training in an attempt to correlate manual dexterity with technical success in the profession. There has been no general agreement about the results and debate continues about the reliability and predictive nature of the tests [3,7,10,12,13]. An objective comparison of manual dexterity in physicians and surgeons was carried out and analysis of the data showed no significant difference in dexterity between medical and surgical residents [11].

This would suggest that physicians with no surgical skills had manual dexterity ratings equivalent to those of their surgical colleagues and indicate that manual dexterity is not the primary determinant of surgical skills. A further study by Schueneman et al found that pure psycho-motor skill was not the major factor in distinguishing the proficient surgical performance from the mediocre [9].

Attempts to set up a series of psycho-motor tests based on assessing established surgeons have so far failed to identify the type and extent of tests required (personal communication). Some direction may be obtained by looking at other disciplines such as musicians. After a number of assessments taking into account exercise prior to performance, handedness, visual acuity and arousal tests, manual dexterity was regarded as too simplistic an assessment to determine ability in the higher level task of playing a musical instrument [1,2,4,5].

If a test is to be set-up to determine manual dexterity in surgery, then a definition of the end point needs to be made. M. Salcmann produced an apt description saying that "in surgery, there is an illusion created of effortless grace and efficiency based on a lifetime of study and enforced discipline" [8]. We, therefore, need an assessment of dexterity which equates with not only clinical competence but also the retention of that competence. The assessment would have to be relevant, reliable, validated and beyond reproach as jobs and livelihood would be affected. We would expect to know that the appropriate skills were present on the day of assessment but we would require an additional factor to indicate the likely persistence of those skills.

If we are to examine manual skills, we need to be aware of some factors that may influence the performance of the candidate. The correct use of the hands, the effect of tremor, the appropriate instrument, spatial awareness, organisation and control of the environment.

The hands are, of course, paramount in the assessment. Trainees would need to be aware of the fact that the hand has two grips, one powerful and the other delicate [6]. In the powerful grip mobility is at the wrist joint or more closer to the trunk. The movement is powerful and though it can be controlled to a remarkable degree, it is not suitable for small movements. This is the type of grip used for retraction. The more delicate grip is with the fingertips with mobility at the wrist or by coordinated movements of the thumb and fingers. This is the grip required using micro-instruments though an additional factor – tremor – may come into play. Both grips may be used simultaneously in the same hand – holding an instrument and tying a knot – and both would need to be assessed in any test of dexterity.

It is normal to have tremor in the unsupported hand. There are a number of determining causes that can increase tremor, these include tiredness, lack of support of the limb, psychological factors and stimulants such as caffeine, alcohol and tobacco. Tremor,

of course, can be reduced by support and trainees need to be aware of this practical fact and develop methods of controlling their tremor. In assessing dexterity tremor probably should be considered, but it would increase the complexity of any assessment.

In determining dexterity the trainee needs to be using the correct instrument for any particular surgical task. Trainees should be familiar with their instruments and this implies exposure and specific training to develop skills. Experience increases the appreciation of the importance of the correct instrument selection based on design, shape, size, weight and, of course, appearance. Surgeons using either the wrong tool or an unusual instrument can be made to look clumsy.

Other actions can lead to a lessening of dexterity. Poor positioning of the patient and the microscope with poor organisation and lack of control of the intra-operative environment can result in a loss of fluency of movement and dexterity.

Lack of spatial awareness can affect manual skills. It is usual for the trainees during their initial training to experience difficulty in appreciating the relationship of deep seated pathology to the surrounding structures particularly when using the microscope. Over a period of time with the appropriate training their sense of spatial awareness will develop and improve. The appreciation of anatomy in 3-D is a fundamental requirement for the Neurosurgeon and any assessment of manual skills related to competence should include this factor.

Can these and other factors be organised into a test of dexterity?

Should we attempt to design a test (usually stress related) to assess an end organ function (the hand) to determine competence in performing a calculated risk strategy (an operation) in a highly organised technical environment (a theatre) on a complex articulate, sophisticated animal (man)? If we were to design a test to just assess dexterity, then I would suggest we are starting from the wrong end and looking in the wrong direction.

We should attempt to establish the position of manual skills is the context of training the competent surgeon. In this attempt Wood Jones's comment that "in man this manipulative function (dexterity) achieves its most complicated state because of an undifferentiated hand and a highly developed part of the brain controlling it" is important [14]. The hand can carry out any function but dexterity is acquired at least in part and sometimes wholly by mental training. This opinion is further strengthened by the observation that surgery is nothing but trained and organised common sense. It, therefore, needs to be argued that a holistic approach is required in the selection and training of future neurosurgeons.

Clearly we can only select from those who want to do neurosurgery and while important qualities such as determination, commitment, humility, patience and a sense of humour are important, I would also add the need to be a good observer and to have more than a modicum of common sense. Surgical training needs to be right, and this will be the result in trainees thinking in the right way. In good surgical training there will be a transfer of competence from trainer to trainee and part of this transfer should be the necessary manual skills. If the training has been right, this will lead to the development of leadership, organisation skills, discipline and good judgement with the trainee recognising their own limitations.

In order to ensure an appropriate background for this holistic approach, there needs to be regular and repeated assessment of training competence. Training programmes need to define the type of surgeon they would wish to develop. This will depend on the spectrum of pathology and expertise that is available in the training unit as well as the amount of protected teaching time and focused exposure granted to the trainee. Over and above this, trainer commitment is of paramount importance.

This paper has attempted to consider the question of whether manual skills in surgical training can defined or measured. I would suggest that manual skills for surgical tasks need to be defined within the overall context of a training programme and that the

measuring of manual skills, were it possible, are unlikely to indicate competence.

References

1. Annett M, Kilshaw D (1983) Estimating the parameters of the distribution of L-R differences in male and females. Br J Psychol 74:253–268
2. Elliott M, Waldron JR, Anton BS (1995) Effects of exercise on dexterity. Percept Mot Skills 80:883–889
3. Graham JW (1972) Substitution of perceptional motor ability test for chalk carving in Dental Admission Testing Program. J Dent Educ 36:9–14
4. Hancock PT, Hockley HF (1984) The effects of stress on human performance. Fearon Pitman, Belmont CA
5. Neiss R (1988) Reconceptualying arousal: psychological states in motor performance. Psychol Bull 103:345–366
6. Patkin M (1965) The hand has two grips: an aspect of surgical dexterity. Lancet i:1384
7. Peterson S (1974) The ADA chalk Carving test. J Dent Educ 38:11–15
8. Salcman M (1992) The education of a neurosurgery: the two cultures revisited. Neurosurgery 31:686–692
9. Schueneman AL, Pickleman J, Hesslein R, et al (1984) Neuropyscholoigcal predictors of operative skill among general surgery residents. Surgery 96:288–295
10. Smith BG (1976) The value of tests of spatial and psychomotor ability in selecting dental students. Br Dent J 141:150–154
11. Squire D, Giachind AA, Profitt AW, et al (1989) Objective comparison of manual dexterity in physicians and surgeons. Can J Surg 32:467–470
12. Thompson GW, Ahlawat K, Buie R (1979) Evaluation of the dental aptitude test components as predictors for dental school performance. Can Dent Assoc J 45:407–409
13. Ulmer FC (1976) The wax carving test. Quintessence Dent Technol 1:71–74
14. Wood Jones F (1949) Principles of anatomy as seen in the hand. Balliere, Tindall & Cox, London

Correspondence: G. Neil-Dwyer, MS FRCS, Wessex Neurological Centre, Southampton University Hospitals, Tremona Road, Southampton, Hants, S016 6YD, United Kingdom

Acta Neurochir (1997) [Suppl] 69:30–32

How many Residents Should we Train? The USA Experience

R. H. Patterson Jr.

New York, NY, U.S.A.

Summary

Over the past ten years, an average of 135 residents have entered neurosurgical training in the United States each year. These neurosurgeons-to-be come from about 250 applicants who annually enter the national matching program for neurosurgery. After completing training, they join a pool of practicing neurosurgeons that includes about 3,260 board certified neurosurgeons and an additional 390 practicing neurosurgeons who are still in the certification process. The pool of active neurosurgeons does not increase by 135 surgeons each year since the forces of retirement and death serve to decrease it. Judging by the experience of some large Health Maintenance Organizations, who employ no more neurosurgeons than are necessary to supply their enrolled members, the net result is that the USA has at present about the proper number of neurosurgeons necessary to meet the needs of the country. No one can predict future needs for neurosurgeons with accuracy, and it is safer not to set the number of neurosurgeons based on a guess. We do need to restrict the number of trainees to that number we can train properly. The quality of our neurosurgeons needs to be maintained. Beyond that, the market place, however imperfect, is a better long-term regulator of numbers than any governmental or privately-based committee.

Keywords: Neurosurgical training, Neurosurgical Manpower, United States.

At the present time, about 140 neurosurgeons finish training programs in the USA each year, which is a slight increase from years past. This number is added annually to the present population of practicing neurosurgeons, which includes about 3,260 who are board-certified and in practice, plus approximately 390 individuals who have completed a residency and are awaiting their turn to take the oral examinations and become certified. There is also a small group of neurosurgeons who are practicing but will never become certified. The size of this latter group is dwindling at the present time as hospitals are refusing to give them surgical privileges and payors are refusing to pay them. At the same time a number of neurosurgeons retire from practice each year, others die, and a very few have their board certification revoked, usually related to the loss of medical licensure. The net effect is that the number of practicing, board-certified neurosurgeons is increasing very slowly at the present time (Table 1).

The number of neurosurgeons in the USA seems to be about right, though some argue that they are in slight oversupply. That's not to say that the distribution of neurosurgeons is reasonable, because it is not. Some places, such as southern California, seem overpopulated with neurosurgeons, and in other areas there seem to be not enough. The USA has a population of about 280,000,000. Therefore, the ratio of board certified practitioners to population is 1 per 86,000, or, looked at another way, 1.16 per 100,000 population. If all possible practitioners are taken into account, the ratio of neurosurgeons to population is about 1.5 per 100,000. This is higher than in many other industrialized countries, but a case can be made that other countries could use more neurosurgeons if they only provided the gamut of services that neurosurgeons in the USA provide. One capitated health plan in Portland, Oregon, the Kaiser group, employs 1.3 neurosurgeons per 100,000 covered lives, which is not far off the present ratio of neurosurgeons in the USA for the population as a whole [1,2]. Looking at the number of neurosurgeons from the perspective of a training program director, finding a place for the graduates of neurosurgical training programs is never a problem. The demand for new neurosurgeons seems to be high.

How many neurosurgeons should we train? The answer seems simple: train enough to carry the

Table 1. *The Number of Practicing, Board-Certified Neurosurgeons in the United States (Derived from Data Kindly Supplied by the American Board of Neurological Surgeons)*

Year	Number of practicing, board-certified neurosurgeons	change	Annual per cent change
1990	3,017		
1991	3,080	63	2.05
1992	3,135	55	1.75
1993	3,230	95	2.94
1994	3,228	−2	−0.06
1995	3,261	33	1.01
1996	3,267	6	0.18

neurosurgical workload, no more, no less. Here it gets complicated. What is the neurosurgical workload? How many neurosurgeons does it take to carry this workload?

The size of the workload depends on what disorders and operations are in the proper domain of neurosurgery. Does it include extracranial vascular surgery? It does in New York, Boston, Memphis, and many other places but not so in California, where almost all carotid endarterectomies are performed by vascular surgeons. Comparable geographic variations can be observed in peripheral nerve surgery and spinal instrumentation. In some places, epilepsy and functional neurosurgery comprise an important part of neurosurgical practice, but elsewhere these fields are almost completely ignored.

The neurosurgical workload could increase in the future. Change has occurred in other specialties. Cardiac surgery, for example, was at a low ebb in the 1960s. Most of the backlog congenital hearts had been repaired, and the supply of patients with rheumatic valvular disease was drying up. Then the coronary bypass procedure was developed, and the specialty was revitalized. The same could happen in neurosurgery. Suppose a drug perfused into the ventricles would ameliorate Alzheimer's disease? Neurosurgeons would find themselves overwhelmed by calls to implant pumps to deliver the drug.

Even if the scope of neurosurgery stays constant, it might well be that we need more neurosurgeons to carry the same workload. Presently, the average neurosurgeon works 60 hours per week in the USA. In many other countries, the neurosurgical workweek has been curtailed by law and now is as low as 35 hours per week in some places. We are beginning

to see the first signs of this in the USA, where some states have limited the working hours of residents in training. We are also seeing more and more women entering the field, and it is entirely possible that they might want to have more of a life with their family than male neurosurgeons have traditionally sought. Another consideration is that the hassle of practice is on the increase. Neurosurgeons are being sued more often for malpractice. The paper work is exploding, and payors are trying to limit our options in dealing with neurosurgical disorders. The stresses of contemporary practice could lead more neurosurgeons to seek early retirement. The net effect would be a need for more neurosurgeons, not less.

On the other hand, if we still think of neurosurgeons in the mold of Harvey Cushing, a surgeon who only operates on brain tumors and perhaps aneurysms, then we need fewer of us than we have at present. But times have changed; modern neurosurgery is far more than Harvey Cushing could have imagined. No one neurosurgeon can do or even wants to attempt every neurosurgical operation. None of us does spinal instrumentation one day, craniofacial surgery the next, and a procedure for Parkinson's disease the following. We all look for our niche of special competence.

Why should we even worry about the number of neurosurgeons? Why not let the market place determine our needs? There are two prime reasons given for trying to peg the number of neurosurgeons at a reasonable point. The first is that training a neurosurgeon is expensive. Training too many of them is a waste of scarce societal resources at a time when all nations are concerned about the cost of providing health care. The second concern is that if we are overpopulated with neurosurgeons, then the neurosurgeons will not be busy, their surgical skills will rust, and their competence will dwindle. A corollary of this second point is that if neurosurgeons don't have enough to do, then perhaps they will manufacture work and perform some operations of marginal worth. All of these points can be argued. Competence is determined by more than the sheer number of operations performed. Other entities are looking to preserve competence, such as hospital review boards, malpractice lawyers, and state boards of medical licensure. Some cynics have speculated that there is a third, usually unspoken, reason to contain the number of neurosurgeons, which is to preserve neurosurgical income. The argument goes that the more neurosurgeons there are, the smaller will be the slice of the health care pie for each neurosurgeon. This is not much talked about, and its impact is impossible to calculate.

If the numbers are to be regulated, who should do it? I would argue that taking into account all the unknown variables, no person or group can predict the manpower needs for neurosurgery. Therefore, we are better off not to regulate the number of neurosurgeons by trying to guess at future needs. If by any chance a group were delegated by law to set numbers of neurosurgeons to train, that group would have to have broad-based composition since the number of doctors to train is a societal issue that society should decide. The number of neurosurgeons to train is too important to be left to the neurosurgeons. No matter how broadly based, I say that no such group should be formed since no one has the insight to divine the neurosurgical needs of the future.

Though full of inefficiencies, the market place is the best regulator of neurosurgical supply. All organized neurosurgery can reasonably do is to make sure that our neurosurgical training programs are of high quality and that our graduates are good, safe practitioners.

The quality of the training programs is in the province of the Residency Review Committee (RRC). Any group, usually based in a university-affiliated teaching hospital, can apply for a residency training program in neurosurgery. The standards that must be met are set by RRC at a level calculated to provide a safe, competent neurosurgeon at the completion of training. The standards take into account the range and volume of surgery in the institution, the quality of the neurosurgical staff, the academic environment, the evidence of academic productivity, and the availability and quality of the ancillary services. Ancillary services include neuroradiolgy, neurology, neuropathology, the laboratory and library facilities and so on. These standards are applied equally to all programs, both first time appliers and established programs up for periodic review. The result in 1996 was that the 97 approved residency programs were allowed to offer 146 first year residency positions.

The trainee must pass a multiple choice examination, usually taken near the end of the training period. Having passed this written examination and having satisfactorily completed the training program, the neurosurgeon must practice neurosurgery for two years before becoming eligible to take the oral examination given by the American Board of Neurological Surgery (ABNS). A neurosurgeon who passes both examinations then becomes "Board certified." This means that the neurosurgeon has completed a satisfactory period of training and has the knowledge that it takes to be a good neurosurgeon. It does not mean that the neurosurgeon is competent, only that he or she has received good training and has demonstrated command of the knowledge basic to competency. The members of the ABNS believe that no examination can measure neurosurgical competence.

The social environment in which neurosurgeons practice is changing rapidly all over the world. In the USA, the health care system is fast evolving from a cottage industry to big business. Hospitals are forming chains with access to the equity markets. Payors are now large corporations or the government. Patients are bound into large groups, and the contract to deliver their health care is up for bids in the market place. Only the doctors have tended to stay in solo practice or in small groups. This fragmentation has severely limited the doctors' ability to negotiate, and the result is that physicians are experiencing a financial squeeze that will no doubt continue until they find a way to band together and thereby gain some leverage in the negotiation process. For physicians, including neurosurgeons, to negotiate successfully, their numbers must be in reasonable balance with physician need. If there is a big physician oversupply in a medical specialty, then it is difficult to have leverage on the hospital chains and large payors of medical care. Fortunately, in the United States, a reasonable equilibrium exists between supply and demand with respect to neurosurgeons.

References

1. Menken M (1991) The workload of neurosurgeons: implications of the 1987 practice survey in the USA. J Neurol Neurosurg Psychiatry 54:921–924
2. Weiner JP (1994) Forecasting the effects of health reform on US physician workforce requirement. Evidence from HMO staffing patterns. JAMA 272:222–230

Correspondence: R. H. Patterson Jr., M.D., 146 West 57th Street, New York, NY 10019, U.S.A.

Acta Neurochir (1997) [Suppl] 69:33–35

How many Residents Shall we Train? The Netherlands Experience

C. A. F. Tulleken

Department of Neurosurgery, University Hospital Utrecht, Utrecht, The Netherlands

Keywords: Netherlands Experience, Resident Training.

The number of residents to be trained until the beginning of the '80's was fully determined by the manpower needs of the individual neurosurgical center. When that center happened to be a center with training facilities, it appointed a resident in their own program and when that person finished the training, he or she became automatically a staff member.

When the center in need of a neurosurgeon had no training program, the future staff member was trained in one of 6 training centers in Holland and after finishing his residency he moved to the place where he was wanted.

There was a gentlemen's agreement in the Dutch Society of Neurosurgeons, that no one should be trained who was not in advance assured of a staff position in one of the Dutch neurosurgical departments or, in exceptional cases, for a neurosurgical position in a foreign country (Indonesia, Surinam).

This situation existed from the beginning of Dutch neurosurgery (about 1936) until the beginning of the '80's. This very much decentralized way of manpower planning had the advantage of a full employment for trained neurosurgeons, but had the disadvantage of a constant threat of a shortage in manpower. The steady and sometimes accelerated increase in the need for neurosurgical manpower was not accounted for in that way, neither were unexpected changes in the number of neurosurgeons caused by early retirement, death and illness.

For this reason in the '70's and '80's, around 10 neurosurgeons, who were either trained abroad or were trained in Holland with the purpose of a neurosurgical position abroad (Surinam, Indonesia), were appointed in Dutch centers. This quite substantial number proves the inadequacies of the selection system and proves also the efficacy of another mechanism: individuals who wanted at all costs to become a neurosurgeon found a resident position (mostly in Germany) and at the moment of acute manpower shortage in Holland, returned to their native country as a staff member in one of the neurosurgical departments, thus bypassing the Dutch planning system.

During the '80's, when the number of neurosurgeons in Holland had increased from around 20 in the '60's to around 70, the Dutch Society of Neurosurgeons advised its members, who were head of a training program (6), to train no more than 3 residents at a time. It was not required anymore that residents knew in advance where their future job as a neurosurgeon would be, but with this number of trainees (between 1 and 3 per training center) full employment seemed to be ensured because of the retirement of older colleagues and the steadily increasing need for more neurosurgeons (Fig. 1a,b).

It is estimated that in the beginning of the next century a number of between 100 and 110 neurosurgeons will suffice in Holland (population 15.5 million). Although the number of trainees is possibly too small to fill up all vacancies caused by retirement, unplanned early retirement, illness ect., and since the number of 100–110 is a rather conservative estimate, this does not mean that vacancies will result. There is a contingent of about 20! (the exact number is not known) Dutch trainees in Germany, who are all very eager to return to Holland after their training since, because of the huge number of residents trained in Germany, there is no chance for them to settle as a

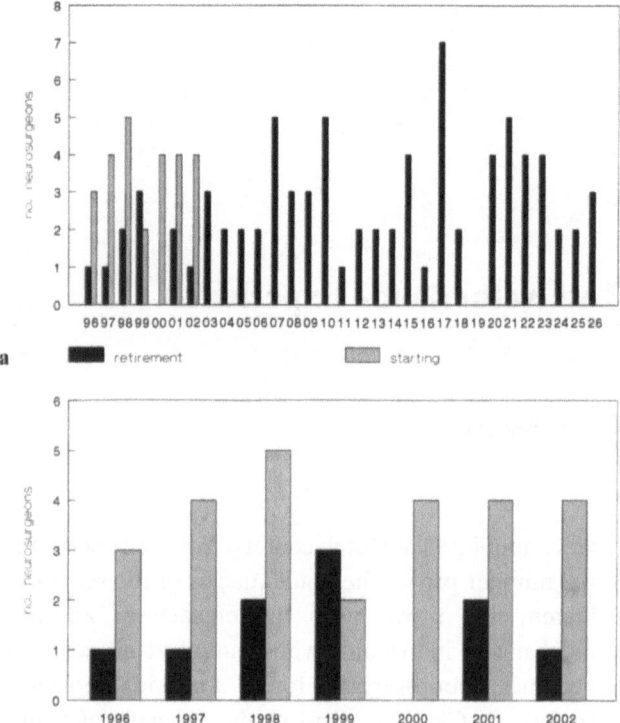

Fig. 1. Manpower planning: neurosurgery Netherlands (**a** 1996–2026, **b** 1996–2002)

neurosurgeon in that country. The problem is that in Holland we have no insight in the quality of training programs abroad. Some of those neurosurgical departments do have an excellent reputation, but the enormous number of trainees (up to 20 in some places) makes it doubtful whether the Dutch trainee in that center will get the opportunity to perform at least the minimum number of neurosurgical procedures that is required in Holland. Other centers in Germany, where Dutch residents are trained, are rather obscure and it is difficult to get information about the quality of their training programs.

In recent years there has been a tendency in Holland to decentralize the planning of the number of trainees again, but quite differently from the early decades of neurosurgery. In early times, as mentioned above, residents were only appointed when there was a vacancy in one of the neurosurgical staffs in Holland. By now some of the heads of the training programs in Holland share the view that the number of trainees could solely be decided by:

– The number and complexity of operations performed in a neurosurgical department with a training program,
– The ratio staff members → residents, which has to be 2:1 in most specialties, as ordained by the Dutch Specialist Organization. For example, in my department at the Academic Hospital Utrecht, there are 8 staff members and 3 (sometimes 4) residents in neurosurgery. The total number of residents is 7, but 3–4 of them are not part of the training program.

Because of the natural turnover and the increasing need for more neurosurgeons in The Netherlands, all trainees in my department will be assured of a staff position as a neurosurgeon somewhere in Holland, but I personally hope that most of them will stay at our department after finishing their training, otherwise we will have a real shortage of manpower.

The Dutch Association of Neurosurgical Residents has a somewhat different opinion about the matter of manpower planning. As may be expected from trainees, who want to operate on as many patients as possible, they are afraid that there will be too many neurosurgeons in the beginning of next century. They do, however, admit that also a shortage of neurosurgeons at that time can not be excluded because of unpredictable factors as early retirement, illness and further increase in the number of neurosurgical interventions (Fig. 2).

They share with their teachers the opinion that the main factor deciding about the number of residents trained is the quality of training. The ideal situation is

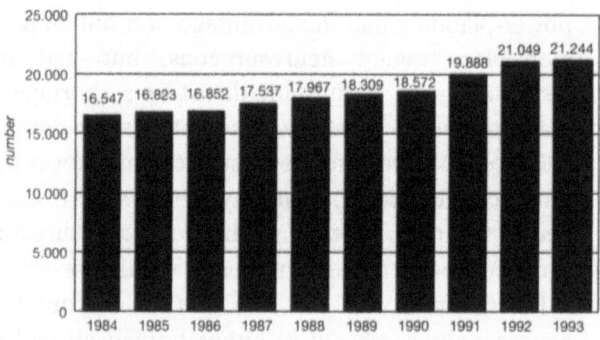

Fig. 2. Number of neurosurgery patients operated (source: LMR)

that for each 2 staff members there is 1 trainee, and furthermore that in a center where 4 residents are trained, at least 1,200 neurosurgical procedures of sufficient complexity are performed.

When the criterium of quality of the training program is the main leading principle an adequate number of residents will be trained, at least in Holland where 7 training programs are in existence nowadays.

Correspondence: Dr. C. A. F. Tulleken, Department of Neurosurgery, University Hospital Utrecht, P.O. Box 85500, NL-3508 GA Utrecht, The Netherlands

Acta Neurochir (1997) [Suppl] 69:36–39

How Many Higher Neurosurgical Trainees Shall We Train in the British Isles?

M. D. M. Shaw

The Walton Centre for Neurology and Neurosurgery NHS Trust, Liverpool, United Kingdom

Summary

In the British Isles there are a small number of neurosurgeons. The number of career trainees has been rigorously controlled over the years, such that there is a sufficient number to satisfy the number of new consultants required as the result of retirement and the creation of new posts. The number of career trainees posts is 89 but the current calculated requirement is for 112 career trainees. In addition overseas trainees come to the British Isles, usually for a specific part of their training.

Keywords: Neurosurgery, trainees, British Isles.

Introduction

In a small speciality such as neurosurgery calculations relating to the number of trainees required, only make sense if the consultant requirements and hence career trainee requirements are considered for the whole of the British Isles because of the interchange between the 5 countries. It is on this basis that the Joint Committee for Higher Surgical Training (representing the Royal Colleges of Surgeons, the Association of Professors of Surgery and the Specialist Surgical Associations in Great Britain and Ireland) and its subcommittee the Specialist Advisory Committee (SAC) in Neurological Surgery has worked when presenting information about the number of career trainees.

Number of Consultants Required

Before considering the number of neurosurgical trainees who should be trained it is necessary to determine how many neurosurgeons are needed for the population which the training programmes serve. In the British Isles we have taken a relatively conservative view of the number of neurosurgeons required, believing that all neurosurgeons should be carrying out major neurosurgery in order to maintain their expertise. This necessarily means that it is impossible for all patients who sustained head injuries requiring admission to hospital to be seen by a neurosurgeon. The Society of British Neurological Surgeons has taken the view that subspecialisation will continue to develop and that it will be necessary for individual neurosurgeons to gain a considerable amount of experience within the subspecialities, e.g. it is considered that a neurosurgeon undertaking the management of aneurysm cases should manage at least 25 cases per year. On this basis, together with some geographical considerations the Society of British Neurological Surgeons, 3 years ago, recommended [4] that there should be 171 neurosurgeons for the population of the British Isles, including Eire.

It follows from these considerations that the objectives of the completed neurosurgical training programme must result in the trainees being capable of:

- Being eligible for consultant appointment in the National Health Service (NHS) as judged by the ability to:
  - practice general neurosurgery competently and independently including the provision of continuity of care for patients
  - practice with special expertise in at least one of the subspecialities and/or research and
- contribute to service and/or academic developments within the speciality.

Initial Trainee Numbers

In the British Isles there are 2 types of higher surgical trainee:

- career who are trainees who have right of residence in the European Union
- overseas or visiting trainees who do not have residency rights in the European Union.

It is important that the number of career trainees does not exceed the number required to fill future consultant posts by any substantial margin. Neurosurgery over many years in the British Isles controlled the number of trainees who were training for appointment within the British Isles. However in the late 80's this role was taken over by official national bodies. In England and Wales as of March 1995 the JPAC (Joint Planning Advisory Committee) allowance for career higher trainees in neurosurgery was 59, of which 32 were at senior registrar level and 27 at registrar level. In the other parts of the British Isles there were similar bodies limiting the number of career posts:

- Scotland: 5 senior registrars and 5 registrars
- North Ireland: one senior registrar and one registrar
- Eire: one senior registrar and 3 registrars

Thus the total number of career trainees in the British Isles as of March 1995 was 75. However, many of us within the Society felt that JPAC had made incorrect assumptions and hence the calculations were wrong. This resulted in too few undergoing career training in neurosurgery and consequently some consultant posts when advertised, only attracted one applicant.

In addition the British Neurosurgical Training Programmes have trained neurosurgeons who plan to practice overseas. These trainees rarely now come for the whole of their training but come for specific purposes e.g. to gain some practical skills such as microvascular surgery or to take the intercollegiate speciality examination in surgical neurology. The number of such posts in a unit is not governed by the official bodies, but by the total number of trainees which the SAC in Neurological Surgery thinks a unit can train and by whether or not a salary can be provided for the trainee.

Future Consultant Requirements

The Society of British Neurological Surgeons, in addition to publishing "Safe Neurosurgery" [4] in which it recommended 171 neurosurgeons for the British Isles, carried out a survey which was completed in early 1994 of the 149 current consultant staff, of whom 118 were in England and Wales, 18 in Scotland, 4 in Northern Ireland and 9 in Eire. The objective of the study was to provide information in order to try to determine future consultant requirements. In the 5 years prior to 1994, 35 consultants had left the NHS, of whom only 7 had reached the age of 65 and 6 were 55 or younger. There were 12 consultants who were aged 60 or more but from 116 respondents currently practising in the NHS or doing non-private neurosurgery in Eire, 14 consultants said they would definitely retire within the next 5 years and 6 indicated they would almost certainly do so. Thus, in the subsequent 5 years British neurosurgery would require at least 25–30 replacement consultants, i.e. 5 or 6 per year. This was the rate at which retirements had been occurring up to that date.

In addition there was a perceived need for a further 41 consultants in the next 5 years to implement the standards set out in "Safe Neurosurgery" [4]. However, unfortunately this report was published just preceding the full understanding of the effects of 3 national documents which have been published concerning the junior doctors, i.e. those in training.

1. Achieving a Balance [3] – which attempts to ensure that the number of trainees will only be equal to the number of consultants required
2. Junior Doctors Hours [5] – which restricted junior doctors to a normal working week of 40 hours, of which at least 4 hours had to be spent in formal education outside the clinical work, and 32 hours on call duty, only 16 of which could be worked and
3. The Calman Report [2] which required the setting up of unified higher professional training programmes in which there would be more formal teaching rather than learning by apprenticeship as had been the case in training programmes to date. The old senior registrar and registrar posts have now been replaced by a new higher training post – the specialist registrar.

It is almost certain that the implementation of the recommendations in these 3 documents will result in a major shift of work from the junior trainees to the consultant staff requiring a further increase in consultant establishment. It was therefore felt reasonable that at least 7 new consultant posts would be generated per year, thus making the total consultant requirement per annum a minimum of 12.

Other Factors Affecting the Number of Trainees Required

The SAC in Neurological Surgery and the Society of British Neurological Surgeons believe that other factors must be taken into consideration if the number of trainees produced is to be sufficient to fill the vacant consultant posts in the future:

1. a) The Calman [2] unified higher training programme in neurosurgery in the British Isles will be 6 years in duration.

   b) At least 6 months will need to be allowed after obtaining the Certificate of Completed Specialist Training (CCST) to obtain a consultant post and hence any calculation of trainees required must therefore be based on the 6 years of the training programme plus this proportion of the 7th year. This is because doctors taking up consultant posts in the British Isles, except Eire, must be on the specialist register held by the General Medical Council as from January 1997. Effectively the only way for a trainee to achieve this is to obtain the CCST. In addition in a small speciality consultant posts do not appear monthly but tend to be grouped and three months notice is required by the employer when leaving a training post.

   c) In addition two thirds of British neurosurgical trainees take time away from clinical training to undertake research. Many obtain a higher degree before becoming accredited. A third of all the trainees spend more than one year doing research and hence it is necessary to add this period of time to their training programme in order to allow them to complete their research. Thus for the purposes of the calculation one third of a year per trainee was added to the total training time, making the total time for the "Calman" training programme 6.8 years.

2. It is expected that there will be a wastage rate amongst career neurosurgical trainees. Currently in the United Kingdom in the superceded training system this is 9% but in the new unified training programme, trainees will be entering the subject with much less experience of surgery in general and neurosurgery in particular. Indeed it will be possible after undertaking a 2/3 year basic training programme in surgery to enter neurosurgery without having any prior experience of neurosurgery.

In these circumstances the wastage rate must increase. Judging from the change in career aspirations amongst the present senior house officer*/registrar groups and those entering programmes in the United States of America, this rate will be at least 30% in the first 2 years. The average drop-out rate was 17% for American residents, when complete 5 year neurosurgical training programmes from 1985–1994 were considered. Therefore a wastage rate of 30% has been accepted for the first 2 years of training and 9% for the remaining 4–8 years. At 14% overall this is not different from the rate for the American programmes.

Actual Number of Career Trainees Required

The SAC in Neurological Surgeon took these factors into account and then decided that the British Isles required:

$(6.8 \times 12^{**})$ plus a wastage rate of 30% for 2 years $+ 9\%$ for 4.8 years = 94 trainees

On a pro rata basis, based on the 161 consultants then in post (April 1995), England and Wales require 75, Scotland 11, Northern Ireland 2 and Eire 6 trainees.

SWAG Calculations

In May 1995 the Chairman and Vice Chairman of the SAC in Neurological Surgery met with SWAG (Specialist Workforce Advisory Group) a subcommittee of the Advisory Group on Medical (and Dental) Education, Training and Staffing (AGMETS) which has recently taken over the function of JPAC at the NHS Executive in Leeds. The Executive have developed a computer model which allows them to determine the number of trainees which are required in England and Wales. The factors entered into this model are:

- Expected consultant retirements as judged by the number retiring per year recently
- Expected consultant expansion which is based upon the proven expansion over the year past
- Duration of higher professional training and
- An expected wastage rate of 15%

---

* Senior house officer is the basic training grade after full registration with the General Medical Council.

** Number of consultant vacancies occurring per year

On this basis in May 1995 SWAG recommended that in England and Wales the number of higher neurosurgical trainees should be raised from 59 to 80, an increase of 21. It was decided that it would not be possible for such a large change to be serviced in one year because there would not be the potential trainees available, nor the number of training slots in the United Kingdom, nor the finance to support them. It was therefore decided to increase the number of trainees by 21 over 3 years, that is to say 7 per year for the next 3 years. Though an increase of 7 has now occurred, when the SAC representatives went to the annual SWAG meeting in May 1996 it was determined that the additional requirement was now 23 trainees. It was again decided to increase the number of trainees over a 3 year period though this increase has not yet been ratified by AGMETS. In June 1996 it was decided following consultation between the Post Graduate Medical Deans and the Royal Colleges that the baseline from which the 1995 and 1996 SWAG calculations should be made for England and Wales was 66 and not 59. Thus the calculated total requirement of career neurosurgical trainees in the British Isles was 112 as opposed to the actual number of 89 career posts.

The aspect of this which gives cause for concern is that the most important variable in the calculation is the number of consultant vacancies (25 in the 12 months May 1995 to April 1996) which result from retirements and the number of new posts created in the previous year. With the recruitment to the service of so many young consultants recently, the number of retirements must reduce, but it will then be too late to correct the number of trainees already in post. I think it is also unlikely that the current expansion of consultant neurosurgeons will continue. It would be encouraging to believe that the expansion from 149 in 1994 to 166 whole time or maximum part-time consultant posts was due to the effects of implementation of the recommendations in "Safe Neurosurgery" [4], but I think in truth that the majority of this increase has been driven by the requirements generated by the junior doctors hours legislation [5]. It is therefore very unlikely that this expansion will continue and that there will be the danger of there being an excessive number of career trainees in the not too distant future.

References

1. Faus P, Colenbrander A (1994) Neurosurgery 35:1172–1182
2. Hospital Doctors: Training for the future (1993) The report of the Working Group on Specialist Medical Training (The Calman Report). Department of Health, UK
3. Hospital Medical Staffing – Achieving a Balance (1987) A report issued on behalf of the UK Health Departments, the Joint Consultants Committee and Chairman of the Regional Health Authorities
4. "Safe Neurosurgery" The Maintenance and Development of High Standards (1993) Society of British Neurological Surgeons
5. The New Deal on Junior Doctors' hours. Department of Health, June 1991 EC (91) 82

Correspondence: M. D. M. Shaw, MA, FRCS, The Walton Centre for Neurology and Neurosurgery NHS Trust, Rice Lane, Liverpool LG 1AE, United Kingdom

Acta Neurochir (1997) [Suppl] 69:40–42

How Many Neurosurgeons Do We Want to Educate in Europe Annually? The Danish Proposal

F. Gjerris and **F. F. Madsen**

University Clinic of Neurosurgery, Rigshospitalet, University of Copenhagen, Copenhagen, Denmark

Summary

The neurosurgical population consists of professors, consultants, specialised senior registrars, and doctors in training (senior registrars, trainees and young doctors to be educated as neurosurgeons). Knowing number and size of the neurosurgical departments in each European country, the number of staff members, the politics of retirement (age, educational level) and the age of every neurosurgeon it is possible to calculate the exact number of trainees needed per year to maintain a state of balance in every single European country. With Denmark as a model we based our assessments partly on a simple calculation model of the exact annual number of neurosurgical trainees or senior registrars and partly used an actuary flow model for calculation. In Denmark with 5 neurosurgical departments, 5.2 mill. population and a retirement age of 70, we have an average of 1–2 newcomers per year and maintain a bulk of 10 senior registrars in education. Thus there will be a balance between intake of newcomers and retirement, of course with some unknown factors as unforeseen dismissal or resignation, death rate among neurosurgeons and transfer to private practice.

Keywords: Education, neurosurgery, number of neurosurgeons calculation model, annual acceptance, Denmark.

Introduction

Many factors influence the education policy in neurosurgery, as for instance size of other specialities, problems in the development or economy of the European national health systems and the superior medical and political policy. There are unpredictable factors such as new developments inside the single speciality, i.e. technical (spine surgery, stereotactic radiosurgery) or biological (molecular biology), which could result in "conservative treatment" rather than in surgery [1]. Subspecialisation within a single speciality may also entail a requirement of neurosurgeons greater than estimated or expected [3,4]. The decreasing weekly working hours for young doctors in training, especially in surgical specialities, observed all over Europe during the last ten years, is also a time prolonging factor in education which has to be taken into consideration.

The neurosurgical population consists of professors, consultants, specialised senior registrars and doctors in training in neurosurgery. This last group comprises senior registrars, trainees and young doctors in introductory positions. Prevalence of neurosurgeons differs in the various European countries, and education policy varies too [2]. A precondition necessary for the calculation of how many neurosurgeons we want to educate annually in Europe or in a single European country is a thorough knowledge of the number of departments, their size and the number of staff members in the single neurosurgical department in each European country, in conjunction with the politics of retirement. Additional information on educational level, retirement age and age of every neurosurgeon on duty renders it possible to calculate the exact number of trainees per year in any country.

The purpose of our work is to try to predict the number of young neurosurgeons to enter training positions in a country per year. With Denmark as a model we based our assessments partly on a simple calculation model of the exact annual number of neurosurgical trainees or senior registrars and partly used an actuary flow model for calculation. The model may also inform about the expected number of unemployed senior registrars, depending on the same factors as mentioned above.

Materials and Methods

Denmark has five neurosurgical departments, a population of 5.2 million and a retirement age of 70. After two basic years, neurosurgical education includes one year of surgery (all kinds), an introductory year of neurosurgery and two years as a trainee in neurosurgery (one year of neurology and one year of neurosurgery), followed by $2\frac{1}{2}$ years as senior registrar in at least two different neurosurgical departments. There is no examination for specialisation.

In the 5 departments we have about 40 lifetime positions (3 professors, 25 consultants, 12 department doctors), about 15 senior registrars, 3 trainees and 6 positions of introduction. In some of the departments a subspecialisation is developing. Unknown factors such as unexpected dismissal, disability or death among neurosurgeons and transfer to private practice should be considered to a small but uncertain degree. Whether we need a surplus production for competitive reasons or desire a job warranty for trainees remains also to be solved before calculation.

Results

Two calculation models are being used:

1. Spread-Sheet Model

The actual working time left for each consultant is calculated. In this model it is possible to incorporate all changes in health system and political influence on the number of consultants needed. The age of each consultant should be known at the time of analysis. Retirement age can then be estimated according to political or individual factors. Hence it is possible to determine very precisely in which periods of time a surplus or deficiency of senior registrars will exist.

2. Actuary Model

Average working years for consultants are estimated as well as the optimal number of years the trainee should be accorded before entering the definite job. This model is suitable for predictions based on overall changes in health systems and training politics. A necessary prerequisite is a fairly large number of senior and junior doctors since the estimated averages in the countries concerned then reflect the actual flow more accurately.

A result of model 1 is shown in Fig. 1, depicting the Danish situation. Retirement age is either 65, 67 or 70 years. If 1 or 2 trainees are accepted annually the number of unemployed specialists can be estimated for each year until 2003. This number represents the trainees needed in case of early retirement as well for some degree of competition between trainees.

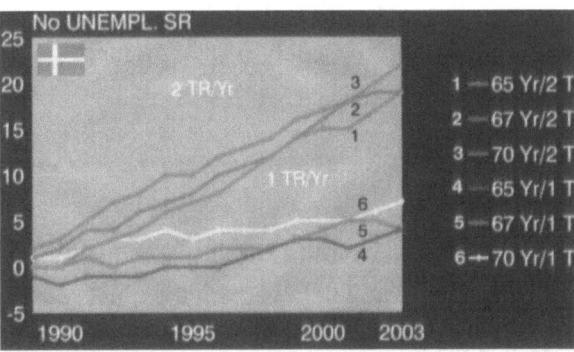

Fig. 1. Danish numbers of unemployed senior registrars, depending on retirement age of consultants (65, 67 and 70 years) and the number of new trainees accepted annually

However, this horror-picture did not occur, because employment rules in the Danish health system were changed in 1993.

In model 2 the formula:

$$\frac{\hat{T}_c}{n_c} = \frac{\hat{T}_t}{n_t} = F$$

expresses the steady state with

n_c = the number of consultants at the present time.
$\hat{T}_c$ = the estimated residual/average working years of consultants.
n_t = the number of senior registrar positions
$\hat{T}_t$ = the estimated average/wanted number of years as trainee.

F can be approximated to the real value at any given time as in model 1 using the formula

$$F = \frac{\sum t_i}{n_c^2}$$

where t_i is the individual residual working time for each consultant.

The exact value F at a given time can then be used in formula 1 to estimate what influence any change might have on the number of consultants, residual time for consultants, number of senior registrars/trainees, and training period. This figure can be used to estimate what will happen starting at a given year. The total number the average working years for consultants can be used to estimate a new or imaginary system.

If we look at the German numbers, it seems that more than 40 newcomers are trained per 80 million population, and if our calculations are correct, in this country only approximately 24 new trainees should be accepted per year.

Conclusion

In Denmark we educate 3 trainees annually for a population of 5.2 million. Based on the above figures we should not educate more than 1.5 trainee per year, if in the future we want to have competition and only a small number of unemployed neurosurgeons. In Europe generally the figures are much higher, and it appears that too many neurosurgeons are educated annually. Further development of calculations and theoretical figures for neurosurgical education is necessary.

References

1. Berney J (1992) The future of neurosurgery. Acta Neurochir (Wien) 116:190–193
2. Izquierdo JM (1990) Programme of neurosurgical education. Acta Neurochir (Wien) 107:171–178
3. Raimondi AJ (1992) The education and identification of a pediatric neurosurgeon. Childs Nerv Syst 8:4–7
4. Ray CD (1991) Clinical neurosurgery as it relates to the lumbar spine: what it does versus what it says. Neurosurgery 29:937–941

Correspondence: F. Gjerris, M.D., D. Sc., University Clinic of Neurosurgery, Rigshospitalet, University of Copenhagen, DK-2100 Copenhagen, Denmark

Acta Neurochir (1997) [Suppl] 69:43–44

How Many Residents Shall We Train? The Iberian Experience

J. Lobo Antunes

Department of Neurosurgery, University of Lisbon, Hospital Santa Maria, Lisboa, Portugal

Summary

The basic features of neurosurgical training in Portugal and Spain are described. Data include demographic characteristics, training requirements and accreditation criteria.

Keywords: Neurosurgical training, Portugal, Spain.

There has been a long tradition of scientific and professional cooperation between Portuguese and Spanish Neurosurgery. In fact, the Portuguese-Spanish Neurosurgical Society formed by A. Lima, V. Marques, S. Obrador, E. Tolosa and A. Ley is the second oldest in Europe. In recent years it became clear that socio-professional conditions were somewhat different in the two countries, and they would be dealt with more effectively if two independent societies were constituted, although it is planned that the old Portuguese-Spanish Society will serve as an umbrella to both organizations, and joint meetings will continue to take place.

Table 1 describes the basic demographic features pertaining to the practice of Neurosurgery in the two countries. The population of Spain is about four times the one of Portugal, and the same proportion stands for the number of neurosurgeons and neurosurgical beds. The number of Spanish residents is, however, just slightly larger than the Portuguese. This may be due to the fact that there is a significant number of foreign trainees or fellows working in Spain, not officially accounted for as residents. It is of interest to emphasize that a growing number of Spanish physicians are presently acquiring postgraduate training in Portugal and I have currently in my service a Spanish resident.

According to the data supplied by the Union Européenne de Medecins Spécialistes (UEMS) concerning the years 1994–1995, there were 17 recognized neurosurgical services in Portugal and 53 in Spain, of which 9 in Portugal and 29 in Spain had training programs.

The number of trainees entering the programs every year varies from 4 to 6 in Portugal and from 15 to 20 in Spain. This number is determined by the Ministries of Health according to the perceived needs of each country. In both countries, the single entering criterion is a multiple choice examination covering all areas of medicine. The highest classified will choose the place to train. There is no interview or any other form of evaluation, and unfortunately family or geographic reasons may dictate the choice, so the services may have to accept trainees not particularly gifted for our specialty. In Portugal, it is the Ministry of Health who determines where training takes place. In Spain, the candidate may choose among one of the services designated for this purpose. The inexistence of an adequate selection process is, in my opinion, one of the major drawbacks of the system.

Duration and characteristics of the training are similar in both countries (Table 2) and follow, in general, the recommendations of the UEMS. In both countries it is required that each resident performs a minimum number of the various surgical procedures as stated in Table 2.

In both countries, there is continuing evaluation throughout the training period. In Portugal, there is also a final examination which consists of curricular evaluation, clinical examination and cognitive testing. The jury is composed of five members, two of them from the service where the resident was trained, and three appointed by the Portuguese

Table 1. *Demographic Data (UEMS 1994)*

	Portugal	Spain
Population (millions)	9,852	39,025
N.° Neurosurgeons	95	360
N.° Residents	42	55
N.° Neuros. Beds	400	1,300
Hab/Bed	103.7	108.4

Table 2. *Training Requirements*

	Portugal*	Spain**
Duration	72 mos.	60 mos + 12 (gen. surg. specialties)
Neurosurgery	48 mos.	52 mos. (***)
Neurology	3 mos.	6 mos.
N.° Cases:		
Brain Tumors	30	30
Spine	50	30
Trauma	30	30
Shunts	20	10
Others	50	50
Peripheral nerves	5	–

*UEMS; **data from 1984 – program flexible; ***includes rotations (Neuroradiology, Neuropathology, etc.)

Medical Association (Ordem dos Médicos). The final certificate is issued by the Ministry of Health. In the past, there was also a Board examination sponsored by the Portuguese Medical Association which was a real "peer review". Unfortunately, for a number of reasons including pressure by the Medical Unions, this was discontinued. In Spain, there is no final examination, and the certificate is issued by the Ministry of Education.

Despite the existence of a final examination in Portugal, it is my opinion that this is an unsatisfactory way of testing the experience of the candidate and

Table 3. *Accreditation Criteria*

	Portugal	Spain
n.° beds	25	40
OR	1 + 1	1 + 1
ICU	yes	yes
Major cases	270	250
Neuroanest.	yes	yes
Neuropath.	yes	yes
Neurorad.	yes	yes

the quality of the training since the examination is quite often a mere bureaucratic formality. In Spain where no final examination is conducted; I was informed that nobody has ever been denied the final diploma.

In Portugal, there is clear opposition from the Medical Unions to the European Examination, which is felt to be against basic professional freedoms, and may create two types of specialists with both political and economical consequences. In Spain, there seems to be also no sympathy for this procedure.

The position of the two countries concerning accreditation of the services is detailed in Table 3. The mechanisms to implement this are however still not fully established. The question of recertification is a matter of great debate, but it is our feeling that the progressive standardization of medical care in Europe will make it indispensable in the near future.

Acknowledgments

I thank Prof. V. Calatayud and E. Ferrer for supplying the data concerning neurosurgical training in Spain.

Correspondence: Prof. J. Lobo Antunes, MD, PhD, Department of Neurosurgery, University of Lisbon, Hospital Santa Maria, P-1600 Lisboa, Portugal

Acta Neurochir (1997) [Suppl] 69:45–46
© Springer-Verlag 1997

Neurosurgical Manpower in France

F. Cohadon

Hospital Pellegrin Tripode, Bordeaux, France

Keywords: Neurosurgical manpower, recruitment, limitation of residency positions.

Neurosurgical Manpower

The neurosurgical manpower has been rather stable in France over the last ten years. A detailed account of the present situation is given in Table 1. The large majority of qualified neurosurgeons are working in public hospitals, mostly in university hospitals (245). A limited number, recently slightly increasing, are working in private hospitals (58). Neurosurgeons in training either from France (45) or from foreign countries (65) form a supplementary group (110).

This figure of 303 qualified French neurosurgeons for a population of 58 million inhabitants corresponds to a proportion of 5,2 neurosurgeons per million people. This number should be referred to the number of neurosurgical beds. In 1975, the number of authorized neurosurgical beds had been fixed to 60 per million inhabitants. In 1992 however, this number was lowered to 40 per million. With some problems in defining exactly what is a "neurosurgical bed", particularly in private hospitals, we can assume that the actual number of available beds is approximately 50–55 per million.

In 1992 a report from the committee of medical administration and neurosurgical standards of the EANS [1] proposed that a desirable standard would be 6 neurosurgeons and 70 neurosurgical beds per million people. France is clearly below these standards. However it seems, that a largely held opinion among both Health Authorities and the community of neurosurgeons is, that the present situation is satisfactory and that neurosurgical manpower and neurosurgical equipments adequately cover the needs of the population.

How Many Neurosurgeons Do We Train?

The number of neurosurgeons in training is stringently limited by the Health Authorities, this being part of a program progressively elaborated in the last 20 years designed in an effort to contain and control medical demography (Table 2).

- The number of students accepted into medical schools is fixed every year by an order signed jointly by the Ministry of Health and the Ministry of Public Education. In 1996, 3,576 students (N1) were accepted in the 27 French medical schools.
- The number of medical students accepted to enter a course of medical speciality after six years of general formation, is similarly fixed. A national competition (concours d'internat) is opened every year offering a limited number of places (N2) (1,110 in 1996) distributed among the medical schools and among the medical specialities.
- 22% of these places are alloted to surgical specialities in general (N3) and among these 2% to neurosurgery (N4). These later percentages are only indicative and may be slightly modified by a national and a regional committee (CNEM, CREM)*, to adjust to any particular situation.
- Only students successful at the internship concours are eligible for training in specialized medicine. Each applicant submits his ordered list of preferences for medical schools within a geographical

*CNEM Commission Nationale des Etudes Médicales; CREM Commission Régionale des Etudes Médicales

Table 1. *Neurosurgical Manpower in France 1996*

Qualified neurosurgeons in:		
– *Public Hospitals* • Professors PU/PH		97
• Consultants		94
• Assistants		54
		245
– *Private Hospitals*		58
Total of qualified neurosurgeons		303
– Residents (DES)		45
– Residents (DIS, AFS, AFSA) from foreign countries		65
Total residents in training		110

DES Diplôme d'Etude Spécialisé, *DIS* Diplôme Inter-universitaire de Spécialisation, *AFS* Attestation de Formation Spécialisée, *AFSA* Attestation de Formation Spécialisée Approfondie

Table 2. *Determining Medical Demography, France 1996*

– Number of students entering medical schools (N1) 3,576	N1 = 3,576
– Number of students entering a cursus of specialized medecine (N2) 1,110	N2 = 1,110
– Number of students entering a residency program in surgical speciality (N3) $\simeq$ 22% de N2 = 250	N3 = 250
– Number of students entering a residency program in neurosurgery N4 $\simeq$ 2% de N3 = 5	N4 = 5

Table 3. *Distribution of Authorized Training Positions Among Various Surgical Specialities (Percentages are Indicative)*

Surgical specialities	
Pediatric surgery	3%
Orthopaedic surgery	8%
Thoracic and cardiovascular surgery	3%
Urologic surgery	6%
Visceral surgery	24%
Gynaecology obstetrics	18%
Neurosurgery	2%
Ophthalmology	13%
ENT surgery	12%
Stomatology	13%

region and for medical specialities. A residency position is finally allocated to him according to his rank of admission and to his list of preferences.

This system implies that a given student highly motivated for neurosurgery may not be accepted because all the allowed residency positions are already attributed, or that, which is even worse, another student may be pushed into neurosurgery because there is no room available in ENT surgery or stomatology,

which were his first choices, these later specialities being highly praised among candidates.

This system, complicated as it may appear, works correctly and provides every year a planned number of neurosurgeons. This number is determined as a percentage of medical manpower as a whole and it reflects the situation of our speciality in medicine at the present time. It leads to maintain this situation and more generally the balance between subpopulations of various medical specialities (see Table 3).

How Many Neurosurgeons Should We Train?

In order to maintain our neurosurgical manpower stable at its level, given a pool of approximately 300 neurosurgeons, with an estimated working life span of 30 years, we should recruit an average of 10 new residents per year. With a residency program of 5 years' duration we should have 50 residents at any given time. Presently we have only 45 (Table 1).

It is the common opinion of the neurosurgical community that this number is too tight allowing no adaptation to unpredictable problems or changes in a given regional group, no adequate coverage of new fields in our speciality, and/or no competition with neighbouring specialities in overlapping fields. The mere replacement of retiring colleagues can become quite problematic. Moreover we anticipate difficulties in the coming years since the age pyramid in French neurosurgery is rather unfavourable with too many practicing neurosurgeons being over their fifties. All neurosurgical authorities do hope that in the next years we will be allowed to substantially increase our recruitment.

Acknowledgements

We wish to acknowledge the help and advices of Prof. J. P. Castel President of the French Society of Neurosurgery, Prof. G. Guy President of the French College of Neurosurgeons, Prof. J.-P. Houtteville President of the French Syndicate of Neurosurgeons, in the preparation of this presentation.

Reference

1. Sindou M, Fodstad H, Imielinski B, Kanpolat Y, Morales F, Pagni G, Unger R, Van Acker RF (1992) Present and Desirable Neurosurgical Standards (Board Certified Neurosurgeons, Beds, Operating Rooms) per Million Population for European Countries. Acta Neurochir 116:96–97

Correspondence: F. Cohadon, Hospital Pellegrin Tripode, 1 Place Amelie Raba Leon, CHU, F-33076 Bordeaux Cedex, France

Acta Neurochir (1997) [Suppl] 69:47–54

How Many Residents Shall We Train – The Situation In Germany

J. Schramm

Department of Neurosurgery, Bonn University Medical Center, Bonn, Federal Republic of Germany

Summary

The situation of training neurosurgeons in Germany is reviewed taking into consideration the current figures of finished residencies, the development in the number of training neurosurgical units in Germany, and the personnel and structure of a neurosurgery unit allowed to train. The jurisdiction for specialist training as well as typical problems encountered in training residents are being discussed. In 1992, 130,364 patients, equivalent to 0.94% of all patients in Germany were treated in 4.792 dedicated neurosurgical beds. A total of 644 working neurosurgeons were registered. Between 1986 and 1993, 349 residents qualified as neurosurgeons, an average of 43.5 per year. 57% of neurosurgical units employ non-trainee junior doctors, 13% have no residents, and 62% of departments trained less than one resident per year on average. Only 57% of units finish residency training always on time and only 79% of major units have full training permission. The figures provided in this article do not substantiate the assumption that we have trained too many specialists in the past. The problems which some residency programmes encounter however do suggest that it could be wise not to continue to train specialists at the same rate as in the past.

Keywords: Resident training, neurosurgery, Germany.

Introduction

The training of a young doctor to the level of a specialist, i.e. a neurosurgeon, is governed by a framework of ideas, government rules, self-imposed rules of the regulatory bodies of the physicians' organizations and last, within the neurosurgical department by local rules, the personality of the person responsible for the training programme, the many senior neurosurgeons involved with training and finally the means and case load available in that unit. Specific national rules and traditions, frequently national laws, regulate all aspects of neurosurgeons' training.

To understand the situation in Germany this article will outline figures and facts concerning the staffing and the personnel structure of neurosurgical departments in this country as well as the legal framework. In the next step, the actual output of qualified neurosurgeons in the recent past is described, then problems with training programmes are briefly reviewed and finally the quite variable attitudes concerning the necessary number of neurosurgeons in a specific society and ways to regulate these numbers will be briefly discussed in the context of experiences from other countries.

Structure of Neurosurgical Services in Germany

The committee on structures and personnel of the German Society of Neurosurgery under the guidance of Rüdiger Lorenz in a thorough review of the personnel structure of neurosurgery in Germany has received replies to a questionnaire by 109 chiefs of neurosurgical departments [1]. In these 109 departments worked 1,313 physicians (Table 1). The average staffing at a non-university department was: one chief, three "Oberärzte" (equivalent to an attending neurosurgeon in the US and to a consultant in Great Britain), 6.6 residents and two junior doctors in training. The average staffing in the university department was as follows: one chief, four "Oberärzte", 8.6 residents and 2.5 junior doctors in training. Roughly at the same time in the 1995 statistical yearbook of the Federal Republic of Germany 644 active neurosurgeons were listed in the year 1992 and according to the 1995 membership roster there were 438 full members (i.e. qualified specialists) of the Deutsche Gesellschaft für Neurochirurgie (German Society of Neurosurgery). In addition the Society had 196 associate members of which approximately

48   J. Schramm

Table 1. *1995 Survey on Personnel Structure* [1]

| 109 | chiefs |
| 1,313 | physicians |

Average non – university department
1 chief, 3 "Oberärzte", 6.6 residents, 2 junior house officers

Average university department
1 chief, 4 "Oberärzte", 9.6 residents, 2.5 junior house officers

644	active neurosurgeons*
438	full members (i.e. specialists)**
196	associate members (i.e. ~125 trainees)**

* 1995 statistical yearbook FRG, figures for year 1992; ** Deutsche Gesellschaft für Neurochirurgie, 1993 membership roster

Table 2. *Neurosurgery in Germany (1992)*

4,792	dedicated neurosurgical beds*	
130,364	patients = 0.94% of all patients	
644	neurosurgeons	
	in free practice	70**
	in hospital	555
	in leading position	106
	with free practice	43
	in public administration	9
	others	10

*Statistical Year Book; **multiple entries possible

60% were junior neurosurgeons in training, the other associate members can be neurosurgeons from abroad or specialists from related disciplines.

The 1994 statistical yearbook further gives the following figures for 1992. For a population of 80 millions there were 4.792 dedicated neurosurgical beds, and 130.364 patients had been taken care of by neurosurgeons. These corresponded to 0.94% of all patients treated in hospitals in Germany. The 644 neurosurgeons were working in free practice (n = 70), in a hospital (n = 555), in leading position (n = 106), and in free practice with hospital affiliation (n = 43), in public administration 9, and other positions 10 (Table 2).

Of the neurosurgical units 25% had between 40 and 50 beds and over 50% had between 41 and 70 beds (Table 3). 52% had their own Intensive care unit (ICU) run by neurosurgeons, and in 52 of 81 hospitals with the major responsibility with the neurosurgeons. In 20% the shift rotation in the ICU was organized with neurosurgeons only. This is different from many other countries. Most of the neurosurgical units run their own *outpatient clinic* with 65% having 1 to 3 doctors fulltime in the outpatient clinic. In these 109 hospitals various numbers of

Table 3. *Personnel + Structure of Neurosurgical Units*

Intensive Care Unit:
Size: 25%: 40–50 beds,   >50%:   41–70 beds
ICU: 52% own ICU;   in 65%   major ICU-responsibility
   20% with shift rota
Outpatient clinic:
65% have 1–3 doctors fulltime
On-call doctors:
in hospital: 1: 38 units,   2: 30 units,   3 or more: 21 units
at home: 1: 80 units,   2: 20 units,   3: 1 unit

from [1]

doctors were working on call in the hospital during the night (see Table 3) and in addition, these hospitals had one to three doctors on call at home.

Junior Doctors and Residents in Neurosurgery

Another speciality of German personnel structure lies in the fact that in the same neurosurgical department two groups of junior doctors may be employed: residents in specialist training and junior doctors not aiming for the specialist degree of a neurosurgeon (Fig. 1). This situation in the year 1992 was evaluated with a questionnaire sent out to the chiefs of neurosurgical units in Germany [2]. Of the 88 responders, 11 departments had not a single resident in training, 77 departments had between 1 and 14 residents. In addition, 52 departments employed junior doctors not in training, whereas 36 departments did not have junior doctors in the residency programme. A small minority of 4 had only 1 resident in training. Fiftyfive percent of departments had between 2 and 5 residents in training in the period evaluated. Considering the fact that the residency training for neurosurgery lasts for 6 years, a department that trains one resident per year should have 6 residents in training in any given period of analysis. Of the 77 departments that trained residents at all 77% (n = 60) trained a maximum of 1 resident per year and 62% of those (n = 48) trained less than 1 resident per year. It is interesting to note, that during the same period of time the number of finished residencies for these 88 units was as follows: In 31 departments 1 resident had finished his training and in 10 units 2 residents had finished their training. Since 17 units train more than 6 residents at a time (equivalent to one completely trained resident per year) but only 10 units had finished more than 1 residency in that year, it follows that there was a relatively high rate of residents not finishing their training period on those units which

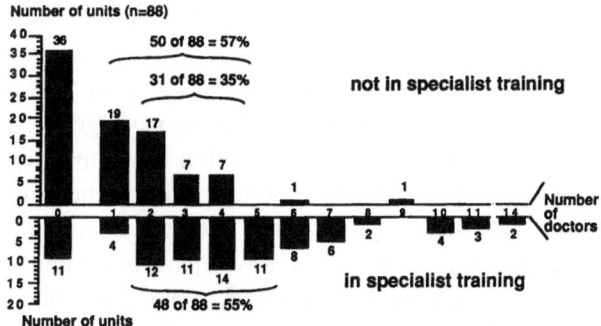

Fig. 1. Number and type of junior doctors employed in 88 departments of neurosurgery. Two main groups are formed, junior doctors in specialist training (bottom half) and junior doctors not in specialist training (upper half)

employed more than one resident per year on average. (Fiftyseven percent of the departments had between 1 and 4 junior doctors who were not in residency training, 35% had between 2 and 4 junior doctors not in residency.)

These incomplete figures for the year 1992 can be supplemented by the official figures from the 16 regional medical certification boards in Germany as outlined in Table 4. As can be seen, the great variations for the regions represent the unequal distribution of neurosurgical departments within Germany. A total of 349 specialists were trained in 8 years, equivalent to an average of 43.5 certified completions of residencies per year for 80 million people.

Regulation of Resident Training

The jurisdiction for specialist training lies completely in the hands of the 16 regional medical boards, i.e. the self-governing bodies of physicians, who are allowed (as many other so-called "free professions") to regulate many aspects of their professional life. All the decisions and bodies of rules established by these medical boards are, however, to be sanctioned by the government, in fact by the interior ministry of the 16 Länder that constitute the Federal Republic. Decisions made on the basis of this rulework can be tested by the administrative courts, i.e. they are debatable, and these decisions can be tested in and be overruled by the administrative public court. In order to achieve a nation-wide uniformity, a general outline of the regional specialist training rules has first been worked out by the committee on specialist training of the federal medial board. This is then voted upon and agreed to by the plenary session of the federal medical board. After that, the 16 regional medical boards may modify the general outlines in less important details and these rulings are then introduced in each of the 16 "Länder" by the regional medical boards. Thus, it is achieved that a specialist who has finished his residency in Bavaria has his degree completely accepted in any of the other 15 "Länder".

The permission to train residents is not automatically granted for each specialist in neurosurgery. This

Table 4. *Number of Completed Residencies with Passed Oral Examinations**

	1986	1987	1988	1989	1990	1991	1992	1993
Baden-Württemberg	0	0	0	4	3	1	0	2
Südbaden	2	1	0	2	1	2	1	4
Bayern	6	2	6	11	7	9	13	5
Berlin	2	3	3	1	2	6	3	1
Brandenburg	0	1	0	0	1	0	1	0
Bremen	2	1	1	3	1	1	4	1
Hamburg	1	0	1	1	1	2	2	2
Hessen	0	7	3	2	6	2	2	5
Mecklenburg	0	0	0	0	0	0	0	0
Niedersachsen	4	1	1	5	6	4	5	5
Nordrhein	6	8	10	9	12	7	8	8
Nord-Württemberg	1	1	2	1	1	0	1	2
Rheinland-Pfalz	3	2	0	5	3	2	0	2
Saarland	3	2	1	0	2	0	1	1
Sachsen-Anhalt	0	0	0	0	0	3	0	0
Sachsen	0	0	0	0	2	0	0	0
Schleswig-Holstein	1	1	1	0	0	1	5	0
Thüringen	0	0	0	0	0	0	0	0
Westfalen-Lippe	5	2	5	6	6	5	9	5
Sum 349	36	32	34	50	54	45	55	43

*Data collected by the author from the 16 regional specialist training certification committees in Germany

right is granted usually to the chief of a department following his application at the Specialist Training and Certification Committee of the Regional Medical Board. The applicant must give detailed information about the capacity of his department, patient numbers, operative figures, affiliation with other specialities etc. He will then be granted the right to teach residents for the full training period of 6 years, or if not all prequisites are fulfilled for a shorter period of time, e.g. 2, 3 or 4 years. Thus, 31 of 35 university departments had full permission for specialist training, 23 of 32 public hospital departments and 12 of 16 health and charity organization hospitals [1].

In daily practice the actual education and training of the residents is, of course, in the hands of all senior staff members of that department. The major responsibility for training may be delegated to one senior staff member of that department for the sake of daily practice, however, only the chief is officially responsible for specialist training and he is the one, who will write the certificate of work for the resident that he will have to submit to the regional specialist training and certification committee at the end of his training period, to be admitted for the final oral examination.

If resident training is looked upon under the aspect of "how many shall we train" it is interesting to analyze who has influence on the number of residents and which facts govern the number of residents. Apart from the well-known factors like the work load and the extent of subspecialization there are specific German aspects that need to be mentioned: since the start in 1996 we have a new law governing working time regulations (Arbeitszeitgesetz), which makes it a legal obligation to send a doctor home the next morning after having been on call, provided that he did not have the opportunity to sleep at least 5 hours.

The next important aspect are certain high court decisions governing the standard of care, where the decision that any operation has to be done with "the standard of a fully qualified specialist" has the most influence on training and working conditions in daily practice. The major impact of this ruling was that for any given operation (be it a burrhole, a chronic subdural hematoma, or even the splitting of a subcutaneous carbuncle) a fully qualified specialist has to be present in the OR. The important consequence of this is that during the night residents are still allowed to operate on their own, but a certified specialist has to come into the hospital. For the chief of a training programme this means that he must have enough fully qualified specialists in his service at all times to ensure that during all periods of the year he can maintain a rota of attending neurosurgeons. In the worst case scenario an attending may have to go into the hospital during a 24 hour shift on the weekend supervising 3 burrholes, the evacuation of 2 subdural hematomas, the removal of an acute lumbar disc plus an acute epidural hematoma, even though the resident on call in that shift is only 6 weeks away from finishing his residency and may already have done a multiple of the number of operations that are required of that particular type to fulfill the requirements. The residency programme chief's decisions are also influenced heavily by the labour laws and by the university laws. It needs to be mentioned here that the universities in Germany nearly all are state-owned universities. Since education belongs to the prime tasks of the 16 "Länder" each of the 16 "Länder" has passed university law, in which many aspects of university life are regulated, especially types of contract, and most important, the duration of working contracts. The federal labour laws not only regulate working time, the handling of sickness benefits but also they regulate the conditions under which a working contract can not be prolonged or may occasionally be ended prematurely.

Since the rules for residency training, set out by the medical regional specialist training and certification committees, also include experience with neurological, neurophysiological and neuroradiological examination techniques as well as the accumulation of a certain number of operations, these conditions alone frequently influence the action radius of the programme chief. Considering the question of "how many shall we train", let us look at who has direct influence on the number of trainees. Taking into account the framework of rules and factual necessities it is only the chief of the training programme who decides on which junior doctor is going to be employed and whether he will enter the residency training programme. Also, he selects junior doctors for a 1 or 2 years period, who later will specialize in neurology, orthopedic surgery, anesthesy or neuropathology. Quite specifically the following institutions have no direct influence on the number of trainees in a department of neurosurgery: the Federal Government, the German Society of Neurosurgery, the Regional Medical Board Certification Committee, the Federal Medical Board, and the

Administrative Director of the University Department. The hospital administration only regulates how many doctors work in a department but they do not interfere with the decision who is going to be trained and who is working as a non-specialist junior doctor. The Regional Medical Board Certification Committee only certifies a training programme but it does not specify how many residents can be trained. This is not necessary, since the prerequisites for an individual's training are put down in form of a list of operations and certain duties that must have been fulfilled when the resident applies for his final oral examination. In practice this means, that in a very big department with many operations you can train a high number of residents provided you are able to give them all what they need to fulfill the requirements.

Problems of Training Progammes

In a survey performed by the author in 1992 as the chairman of the Training Committee of the German Society of Neurosurgery 83 training programmes' chiefs responded to a questionnaire inquiring about problems with the training programme (Table 5).

Table 5. *Problems with Training Programmes*

A. Numeric Requirements of Catalogue of Operations (n = 83)

no problems		47
problems	with	
	tumors	21
	discs	1
	spinal cases	2
	peripheral nerves	13
	hydrocephalus + cer. malform.	8
	cerebral trauma	8
no response		5

B. Reasons for Prolonged Surgical Training (n = 38)

Lack of specific patients	5
Personal conviction that certain things cannot be taught adequately during the 6 years	14
Organisatory or personnel shortcomings not under the influence of chief	19
(48 not valid / no reply)	

C. Duration of Training (n = 77)

Residency training finished after 6 years as a rule	46	(57%)
occasionally over 6 years	16	
mostly over 6 years	9	33 (43%)
usually over 6 years	8	
No reply	11	

Eighty-three responded concerning problems with numeric requirements of the operation catalogue. Fourtyseven of 83 had no problems to provide their residents with all required operations in time. In twenty-one departments were problems with brain tumors, in one there were problems with lumbar discs, in two were problems with spinal cases and in 13 were problems with peripheral nerves, 8 had problems with hydrocephalus and cerebral malformations and 8 had problems with cerebral trauma. The reasons for prolonged surgical training (as answered by 38 units) were as follows: lack of specific patients in 5 departments. Fourteen programm chiefs were convinced that certain things cannot be taught adequately during the residency period of 6 years. In 19 departments there were organisatory or personnel shortcomings not under the influence of the chief of the training programme. The latter reasons most likely refer to the many requirements for specialist training asking for example for certain numbers of technical examinations to be done. Another reason may be regional specialisations with certain types of operations primarily being done by other specialists nearby due to historical or local reasons. A typical example for that would be a neurosurgical unit where due to regional specifics peripheral nerves are mostly done by hand surgeons.

Despite the above mentioned problems 46 of 77 responders mentioned that they finished a residency within the required minimum of 6 years as a rule (57% of all responding departments). Sixteen units needed occasionally more than 6 years, 9 units needed mostly over 6 years and eight usually over 6 years [2]. This means that 43% of responding units to various degrees need more than 6 years.

Discussion

The figures quoted in this article were acquired in the years 1992, 1993, and 1995 from various surveys by the chairmen of the training committee and the committee on structures and personnel, as well as from the statistical yearbook of the Federal Republic. Although the data were not obtained from totally congruent time periods they are pretty informative. The questionnaires were not answered by all chiefs of departments, however, they represent the vast majority.

The key figures related to training of neurosurgical specialists are summarized in Table 6.

Table 6. *Key Figures on Specialist Training in Neurosurgery in Germany*

644	working neurosurgeons
43.5	new specialists per year (completed residencies)
57%	of units employ non-trainee junior doctors
35%	of units employ two or more junior non-trainees
13%	have no trainees
55%	have 2 to 5 trainees
18%	have 6 to 8 trainees
79%	of major units have full training permission
57%	of units finish training always on time

Table 7. *Relationship between Number of Operations and Completed Residencies*

	1988 →	1993	Difference per doctor	Difference per unit
New specialists	+241			
No. of OPs / doctor				
University	92.3	90.6	−1.7	−21.4
Public hosp.	122.6	120.9	−1.7	−28.9
Other hosp.	153.0	161.5	+7.6	+129.9

The discussions during the past frequently centered around the hypothesis (subjective and hardly to verify): we train too many neurosurgeons. The question may be approached by examining the impact of the new specialists added to the system upon number of operations. According to Table 4, 241 new specialists finished their training between 1988 and 1993. Since the number of operations done in the various types of neurosurgical departments is known [1] the average number of operations per doctor can be calculated. The average number of operations at university departments declined by 1.7 per year, in the public hospitals also by 1.7, but increased by 7.5 per doctor in the other hospitals (Table 7). So the "damage" per doctor is either small or nil. Keeping the number of doctors per university department in mind as described above (17 doctors per department), despite the introduction of 241 new specialist neurosurgeons into the system, the number of operations per university department went down by only 29 cases per year. In the other hospital types 11.5 doctors were employed on average and the number of operations in the public hospitals thus decreased by 29 per year. On the other hand the "other hospitals" increased their operations by 129.9 per year. Thus, the facts speak for a steady recruitment of patients into the neurosurgeons' community with a steady net increase of operations.

In the United States with 4,360 Board certified neurosurgeons, equivalent to 1.74 Board certified neurosurgeons per 100,000 people, the relation is quite different from the Federal Republic of Germany where 644 neurosurgeons are available for 80 million people, equivalent to 0.805 per 100,000 people. As can be seen in many articles on this issue, there is a big variation of the number of neurosurgeons throughout the various countries. The question therefore arises who is in a position to define the optimal number of neurosurgeons in a society. If one looks at it from the possible points of view one will realize that the definition of the optimal number of trainees comes under the influence of various interests. You will have quite different answers when you ask the organizations who have to provide the money for health care, or when you ask the official doctors' organizations or when you ask the government.

A similar divergent opinion exists among the neurosurgical community. The attitude of the residents will be quite different from those already working in free practice, which again will be quite different from the chiefs of the training departments. It is quite obvious that the answers you obtain if you ask the diverse interest groups are not only ruled by the supreme demand, namely the provision of optimal neurosurgical care to the community, but also by personal interests. This is evenly true for the government or the health care providers: when looking at the development in countries like New Zealand, Canada, Sweden, the Netherlands, Great Britain and now Germany, it seems that they are not necessarily interested in an *optimal* patient care, but rather in an *adequate* patient care.

This article does not try to find a definite answer to our question, but rather will concentrate on the point of view of the chief of the training programme. His major responsibility is to provide adequate training in the sense of the local rules for the residents in his department. As we can see from Table 5 not all training programmes in Germany are able to provide adequate training in the planned time-frame. Therefore, it might be wise for the chiefs of those programmes to reduce the number of trainees.

Control or No Control for Number of Specialists

Many arguments can be given for or against control of the number of residents in training (see Table 8). The author's main argument against control is, that it

Table 8

Arguments Against Control
- Who knows the future?
- Did it work elsewhere?
- Control through numbers is bad, quality is better
- Artificial narrowing of base of bell-curve
- Is it not just egoistic
- Why is control good if we do it and bad if the state does it?
- Illogical: Proud to expand the field, not the numbers

Arguments for Control
- Many problems in training programmes
- Responsibility for qualified doctors
- Avoids development of mini-units
- Keeps down number of practicing neurosurgeons
- Less expertise with reduced workload

is illogical to expand the field but not the number of specialists. Another important aspect is the question of whether control has worked in other countries. In the Netherlands there are now 27 residents in training, but 10 residents who qualified abroad, were used to fill vacancies in the country. What kind of figures and facts are necessary to develop an accurate plan? How are we going to compensate for the rate of wastage during the residencies, which can be quite different? The wastage rate in England is said to have been 9% in the past but expected to be 30% due to the change in the education system. In the United States it is said to be 17%. How are we going to calculate the loss rate in the German type of residency training, where it is not infrequent to employ non-specialist junior doctors? Most important of all, precise planning of the final output of completed residencies needs either a correct estimate of the wastage rate or it is based on the assumption that basically every resident who starts his residency can be trained up to the end. From many discussions with the members of the training committee of the EANS I know that in several countries it is very difficult and socially unacceptable to give up training a resident to specialist level because of the subjective opinion of the chief that he is unfit to be a competent neurosurgeon.

What do we know about the future development of our speciality? The number of operations in the Netherlands increased from 16.000 to 21.000 from 1984 to 1993 and I wonder how the planning of residents' numbers accounted for that.

If we artificially reduce the number of residents, we narrow the base of the bell curve which depicts the ability of all the residents in training in a given department or a given country. Since we all thrive to pick out the best candidates, it would be much better for the speciality, if the base of the bell curve (the sum of either the residents in one department or in the nation) is broader.

On the other hand, there are strong arguments for control. The major point is, that in many departments the residents see much less cases and turn out to be less well educated and may even be less capable in the actual surgical handcraft. The university chiefs I know well enough had an operative list of between 2.500 and 3.500 operations when they became chairman. If we dilute the workload we may end up with people becoming chief with less than 1.000 operations. This is only possible if we accept that the chief is a subspecialist in his field right from the beginning. But exactly such countries, where the numbers are down-regulated by health authorities, usually have such small units that they cannot afford to only employ subspecialists. Another important factor is the remuneration of neurosurgical specialists. If the proportion of private patients is high, as for instance in the United States, more subspecialists may achieve a good income with lower numbers of neurosurgical procedures per year.

The most important and serious argument for control is to maintain a high quality of the residents and the training programmes. If the problems in the training programmes become more frequent, and due to the steady increase in the requirements for specialist certification they are likely to increase, it may be wise to mildly reduce the number of training positions. Another point is that with increasing numbers of neurosurgeons working in free practice with beds in an affiliated hospital, the danger of too liberal indication for surgery is increasing. Undoubtedly there is a propensity to jump for modern treatment modalities, eagerly picked up by the media and pushed by some neurosurgeons (also in many other specialities). Such techniques in danger of being abused by practising specialists trying to increase their workload have in the past been Chymopaine treatment of lumbar disc or endoscopic surgery of lumbar discs. Politicians do know that, and in some countries they have reacted accordingly, like in Canada where the government now regulates the number of trainees. According to a personal information by Villemure, the number of neurosurgeons in the Canadian Province he is working in has remarkably been reduced by this measure in the last 20 years.

To me a regulation is more attractive if we impose quality measures instead of regulating by numbers only.

It is the author's opinion that in the past we have not trained too many neurosurgeons. There is some evidence that a number of departments have already decided, not to train too many neurosurgeons and instead employ more non-trainee doctors. The number of neurosurgery departments has increased tremendously from the early seventies (around 40) to the mid-nineties (around 140). During the same time, the number of operations in the big university departments has mostly increased and only recently decreased minimally. At the same time the German Society of Neurosurgery has witnessed that the number of neurosurgeons in free practice, which was zero in the seventies, is now around 70. The income structure in Germany makes it difficult for a neurosurgeon to survive if he is only doing minor surgery in an affiliated hospital and spending most of his time seeing outpatients. The author therefore concludes that the facts outlined in this article do not justify the assumption that we have trained too many neurosurgeons, but there is some evidence that we should not continue to train at the same rate as in the past. A relatively high proportion of training programmes already describe problems with the numeric requirements of the catalogue of operations as well as with finishing the residency training in the minimum period of time. This paper has tried to deliver some facts in order to enable the neurosurgical community to form a more well-founded opinion.

References

1. Lorenz R (1995) Struktur und Personalkommission der Deutschen Gesellschaft für Neurochirurgie (ed). Bericht zur Struktur der Deutschen Gesellschaft für Neurochirurgie, Frankfurt
2. Schramm J (1992) Survey on Neurosurgical Training. Bonn (unpublished data)
3. Statistisches Jahrbuch der Bundesrepublik Deutschland (1994) Wiesbaden

Correspondence: J. Schramm, M.D., Bonn University Medical Center, Department of Neurosurgery, Sigmund-Freud-Strasse 25, D-53105 Bonn, Federal Republic of Germany

Acta Neurochir (1997) [Suppl] 69:55–57

How Many Neurosurgeons Should We Train? The Japanese Experience

K. Takakura

Department of Neurosurgery, Tokyo Women's Medical College, Tokyo, Japan

Keywords: Neurosurgeons in Japan, specific activities of neurosurgeons, statistical prediction of needs.

Introduction

In 1995 we had about 6,500 neurosurgeons for a population of 125 million in Japan. The number of neurosurgeons per population is currently the largest of all countries in the world. In order to raise the clinical standard of neurosurgery for the benefit of the patients, it is necessary to make several actions to stabilize urgently the appropriate numbers of neurosurgeons in our country. It is considered to be worthwhile to present to the neurosurgeons in many countries the statistical data of the manpower and activities of neurosurgeons and problems regarding the medical and health care systems in Japan, which have a different medical, social and economical environment. In this paper, I would like to present the statistical data of neurosurgeons, the background of the current medical and health care problems and a proposal for solving the current situation in our country.

Statistical Data

In 1995 there were 6,475 members registered in the Japanese Neurosurgical Society including 108 honorary and foreign members. On the other hand, the total number of neurosurgeons presently working in the neurosurgical clinics was estimated at about 4,500 in 1995. The annually registered number of neurosurgeons working in the hospitals certified by the Japanese Neurosurgical Society is shown in Table 1. The number of board certified neurosurgeons working in the Society certified hospitals in 1981 was 1,037 and increased to 2,964 in 1994. During the same period, the number of non-board certified neurosurgeons was 1,287 in 1981 and increased slightly to 1,365 in 1994. The total number of members registered in the Japan Neurosurgical Society in 1995 was 3,884 board-certified and 2,483 non-board certified neurosurgeons. The discrepancy of the number of neurosurgeons in 1994 and 1995 is explained by the fact that approximately 700 board certified neurosurgeons are working in non neurosurgical clinics, some research institutions or non clinical services. Of 4,500 neurosurgeons currently registered in the neurosurgical clinics, it is thought that about 500 neurosurgeons are performing administrative or research work rather than clinical activities. Therefore it is reasonably estimated that roughly 4,000 neurosurgeons are working today in active neurosurgical services for a 125 million population in Japan, which is approximately one neurosurgeon per 31,000 inhabitants.

Regarding the number of neurosurgical clinics in Japan, there were 302 clinics in 1981, increasing to 998 in 1994. There are 80 medical schools, 191 large hospitals (Category A Neurosurgical Clinics) which can train young neurosurgeons independently and 727 small neurosurgical clinics (Category C) which can train neurosurgeons cooperatively with some major clinics belonging to category A. The total number of neurosurgical operations were 55,117 in 1981, of which 8,559 were major brain tumor operations and 9,557 were major cerebrovascular operations, such as aneurysmal clipping or removal of arteriovenous malformations. The total number of operations increased to 129,314 (19,001 brain tumors and

Table 1. *Number of Neurosurgeons and Neurosurgical Operations in Neurosurgical Clinics Certified by the Japanese Neurosurgical Society*

	1981	1985	1990	1994
Board Certified NS	1,037	1,487	2,276	2,964
Non-Board Certified NS	1,287	1,660	1,636	1,365
Total number of NS	2,324	3,147	3,912	4,329
Total number of oper.	55,117	83,953	109,182	129,314
Brain Tumor	8,559	11,806	16,501	19,001
Cerebrovascular Disease	9,575	14,520	18,382	22,698

NS neurosurgeons; total number of operation includes minor operations such as shunting procedures

Table 2. *Population of the Aged People*

	Age			
	65<		75<	
1992	16 million	(13%)*	6 million	(5%)
2000	22	(17%)	9	(7%)
2010	28	(21%)	13	(10%)
2020	33	(26%)	16	(13%)

*percent of total population

22,698 cerebrovascular diseases) in 1994. Thus, increase has roughly doubled in 10 years. Therefore we can estimate that 4,000 neurosurgeons are doing 130,000 operations annually which means 33 operations per one neurosurgeon.

Background Statistics of Health and Welfare in Japan

The population of Japan was about 125 million in 1995, of which 1,187,067 births and 922,062 deaths (net increase of 256,005) were recorded. Birth rate was 9.5 per 1,000 and is constantly decreasing. The population is estimated to reach the maximum plateau of approximately 127 million before the year 2,005 and then will gradually decrease. Average life expectancy at birth was about 83 years for females and 78 years for males in 1995, compared to 54 years for females and 50 years for males in 1947. The three major causes of death were cancer (28.5%), cerebrovascular diseases (15.9%) and heart diseases (15.1%) in 1995. In 1947 they were tuberculosis (200 per 100,000 population), cerebrovascular diseases (130), cancer (80) and heart diseases (80). During the past 50 years, the death rate of tuberculosis has decreased to less than 0.1% of total deaths, while it increased by more than 200 per 100,000 population for cancer and more than 90 for heart diseases.

Death rate of stroke reached a maximum plateau of 170 per 100,000 population in 1970 and then decreased gradually to about 90 per 100,000 population in 1994. The sharp decrease of the death rate of stroke is considered to be due to the improved health care system for adults to prevent hypertension, obesity, etc., and health education for daily nutrition to decrease sodium, fatty foods uptake, etc.

The current major problem of population in Japan is the rapid increase of the aged people. The number of aged people over 65 years was about 16 million (13% of the total population) and over 75 years was 6 million (5%) in 1992 (Table 2). The number of aged people over 65 years will increase to 22 million in the year 2,000. In 1995, 0.7 million aged people were bed ridden and one million people were thought to be in the mental state of dementia. It is estimated that the number will increase to one million and 1.5 million respectively in the year 2,000. Stroke is obviously one of the major disorders for those aged people requiring medical management and health care.

Activities of Neurosurgeons in Japan

Japanese neurosurgeons are mostly taking care of all patients, as in other countries in the world. Surgery of brain tumors, cerebrovascular diseases, head injuries, anomalies such as congenital hydrocephalus and functional neurosurgery are their major activities. The role of neurosurgeons in Japan is, however, historically slightly different from other countries. Firstly, spine surgery in the past was mainly done by orthopedic surgeons, but there is a tendency that more and more patients are now managed by neurosurgeons. Secondly, most of the stroke patients are being taken care of by neurosurgeons. Even patients with a small intracerebral hemorrhage or an infarction are rather treated by neurosurgeons than neurologists. One of the reasons is that in Japan the number of neurologists is less than the number of neurosurgeons. It is, however, obvious that neurologists are becoming more interested in taking care of stroke patients as compared to a decade ago. Thirdly, the management of brain tumor patients including radiotherapy, chemotherapy and maintenance therapy is mostly done by neurosurgeons. No neurologists are managing brain tumor patients. Finally most endovascular surgery and radiosurgery is done by specialists having experience as neurosurgeons.

Regarding the training system of neurosurgeons, there are guidelines set by the Japanese Neurosurgical Society. Every neurosurgeon must take neurosurgical training for more than 6 years before applying for the board examination. During the 6 years' training period, they must do clinical neurosurgery for more than 3 years. The training of anesthesiology, emergency medicine or basic research work in neuroscience can be included. The applicants must submit reports of 100 cases of personally performed neurosurgical operations. The board examination consists of written and oral examinations. The role and activities of neurosurgeons in Japan seem to be slightly wider as compared to other countries. Young neurosurgeons are encouraged to participate in some basic research work in neurophysiology, neurooncology, neurobiology etc. during their training period. Many neurosurgeons have become specialists of neuroscience as a life time job.

How many Neurosurgeons Should we Train?

The number of neurosurgeons in Japan is obviously overpopulated today. The current number of board certified neurosurgeons is 3,884, of which about 3,200 are active neurosurgeons (Fig. 1). In 1995 there were 265 new members and 80 members retired; thus the

Table 3. *Estimation of Number of Members of Japanese Neurosurgical Society*

	New members	Retirement	Net increase	Total Active BCNS
1995	265	80	+185	3,000
2000	240	150	+90	3,500
2005	200	250	−50	3,600
2010	150	350	−100	3,400

BCNS Board certified neurosurgeon

net increase of active neurosurgeons was 185. It is estimated that the number of board certified neurosurgeons including active and retired members will be about 5,000 in the year 2,000. However the number of applicants for board examination has already reached the maximum plateau and is showing a declining tendency. On the other hand, the number of retired neurosurgeons will increase year by year in the next 20 years. The number of new and retired members is estimated to be the same in the year of 2,002 or 2,003. We can expect 200 new board certified neurosurgeons and 250 retirements, thus the net decrease in the number of active neurosurgeons will be 50 in 2,005 and the net decrease will be 100 in 2,010 (Table 3). Therefore, the overpopulation of neurosurgeons in Japan will gradually improve in the early stage of the 21st century.

We have 80 medical schools and 7,500 students per year. The government has the strict policy not to increase the number of medical schools and the advise to reduce the number of students. It is reasonably suggested that we should train about 150 new graduates from medical schools each year which is approximately 2 graduates per one medical school. Based on the above mentioned statistical data and the current activities of neurosurgeons in Japan, it is predicted that the future manpower of neurosurgeons is not so pessimistic and the problems will be solved spontaneously in the near future.

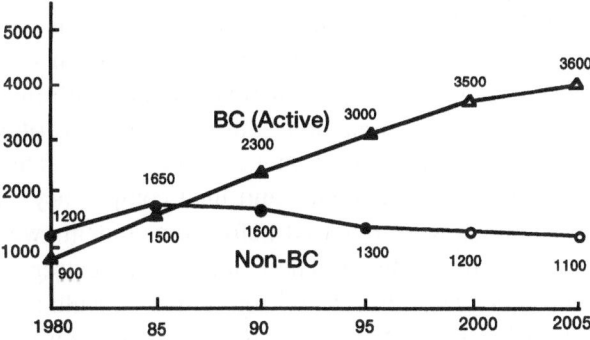

Fig. 1. Number of active board certified neurosurgeons and non-board certified neurosurgeons Japan (Takakura, 1996)

Correspondence: K. Takakura, Department of Neurosurgery, Tokyo Women's Medical College, 8-1, Kawadacho, Shinjukuku, Tokyo 162, Japan

Acta Neurochir (1997) [Suppl] 69:58–64
© Springer-Verlag 1997

Neurosurgical Training at Present and in the Next Century

D. M. Long

Department of Neurosurgery, Johns Hopkins University School of Medicine, Baltimore, Md, U.S.A.

Keywords: Neurosurgical training, Johns Hopkins, competency training.

The Development of the Present Training System

There have been three great advances in medical education implemented in this century and they in turn were dependent upon two important advances which occurred in the last century. The first of these fundamental changes was the development of the concept of the research university. The famous Humboldt Report which appeared in the early part of the 19th century called for research in the university as a part of educational reform, and a new university was established in Berlin based upon the principles embodied in the report. Daniel Coit Gilman was a graduate student at that university and a quarter century later had the opportunity to found the first research university in the United States. Gilman was asked to become the first president of the newly founded Johns Hopkins University, and so based upon the concept of the university as a place for the generation of new knowledge, could develop it. Previously the great universities were simply repositories of knowledge. Now, that this model is universal throughout the world, it is difficult to believe what an enormous change this was. The university system was more than 2,000 years old and it changed very little in a millennium. Our current system, which we all take for granted, is actually barely 100 years old [1,2].

The second major change occurred when Charles Eliott, then President of Harvard, introduced biology into the college curriculum and broadened the curriculum to contain many technical subjects not previously thought to be appropriate for the college or university. The American system of higher education was thus defined quite differently than any that existed in the world, and the opportunity to change medical education was a natural consequence of biology as a legitimate field of study [3].

The greatest advances in medical education in the past 100 years have been: 1) the requirement of college degree and competitive entrance requirements for medical school, 2) education of medical students through practical experience with patients, and 3) the development of the residency concept. All three of these momentous events were a part of the developing new medical school at Johns Hopkins.

When Welch, first Dean of the Johns Hopkins School of Medicine, organized the school, he developed requirements which were unique for the time. A college degree was required for all applicants. Students were selected competitively and women were given an opportunity to compete equally with men. Competitive examinations during training verified learning; clinical education was based upon practical experience with patients; and final competency examinations were required before the students were allowed to graduate. These ideas were extremely controversial. They were rejected by faculties of medicine throughout the world initially. However, Welch and his supporters (who incidentally were four young women who supplied much needed funds for the new school) persisted with the ideas and a quarter of a century later, they were codified in the Flexner Report. This report is the single most important document in modern medical education and was based almost exclusively on the founding principles of the Johns Hopkins School of Medicine.

It is worthwhile reviewing what medical education was like before this time. Most students went to medical school directly from high school or its equivalent. There were medical faculties in some universities, but medicine was generally not a topic of undergraduate or graduate study. Medical faculties had little to do with practicing physicians. There was little selection of medical students and many students entered medical school because of rank, wealth, or family connections. No patient care was required in medical education and surgeons often trained by watching famous surgeons operate in large amphitheaters. For those who were accepted as preceptors of these well-known surgeons, training was indentured servitude. There was no fixed period of training and it was common for individuals to be held as assistants for many years. By contrast, it was also common for a trainee to come for a very short period of time and then go out to practice. No definite surgical experience was required; the public was justly afraid of young surgeons.

The second great step forward was education through patient care. This was actually first suggested by Sydenham in the mid 1700's, but was never implemented. Osler, upon arriving in Baltimore, set about to organize all of the clinical education of the new medical school around patient care. By 1889, this was fundamental in the Johns Hopkins curriculum. However, Osler never introduced true residency training into internal medicine. This was left to Halsted who produced all of our current concepts of residency training between 1885 and 1895. When Harvey Cushing arrived at Johns Hopkins in 1896, it was to join this newly devised surgical training program, and to learn Halstedian surgery based upon careful tissue handling, immaculate hemostasis and anatomical dissection.

What was the Halsted residency? The first principle was a fixed length of training with duties during that training period known in advance. The surgical training was based upon practical care of patients, and an important principle was escalating responsibility as the young surgeon acquired experience and skill. Surgical procedures were learned in the laboratory before proceeding to humans. There was a research experience required. Harvey Cushing actually returned to Baltimore to become the first director of the newly-founded Hunterian laboratory. It is to Cushing and Halsted that we owe our concept of the clinician-scientist. A fundamental principle

throughout was escalating experience in the operating room. The final requirement was a year of supervised practice under the watchful eye of the professor before competency for independent practice was verified.

As we compare what has happened since in residency training, it is worthwhile thinking about the faults indigenous in the Halsted residency. The choice of fixed time periods was arbitrary and meant primarily to eliminate a great evil in medical education at the time, the lack of any defined training requirements. These fixed periods are not necessarily related to the acquisition of skills. All surgeons in the system are assumed to have the same rate of learning. Involvement with patients, while a principle of training, is left to decisions of the professor and faculty, and always is subject to the patient population being treated [4].

How do current requirements in the United States relate to the Halsted residency? Now in neurosurgery the trainee must complete a first year of training in general surgery and related topics. There is a new recommendation from the Board to include three months of neurology in that year. Then 36 months of clinical neurosurgery, both operative and nonoperative, are required, and if neurology has not been a part of the first year, it must be added into subsequent years. A laboratory experience is thought to be desirable, but is not required. Education in neuroradiology and neuropathology is required, but not specified. One of the clinical years has to be the so-called chief residency in which the trainee assumes significant responsibilities for patient care in and out of the operating room. The diversity of subspecialty experience needed is specified and in addition to typical neurosurgery includes pediatric neurosurgical problems, peripheral nerves, functional neurosurgery, pain, spine, and extracranial vascular surgery. A small number of craniotomies per finishing chief resident is a minimum requirement.

The residency system with its obligatory written and oral board requirements and its constant monitoring by the specialty has achieved a generally high level of neurosurgical competency in the United States. Still there are a number of faults with the system that can be improved. It is my view that the experience required in many of the subspecialty areas is too small to ensure that the trainees are competent to deal with complex problems. Exposure and experience are presumed to be the same. If the numbers of patients and operations are present on paper, it is assumed that the resident has played a meaningful role with them. There is no real assessment of competency of care. We do have both an inservice written training examination taken during residency training and an oral examination taken after completion of training and obligatory period of practice. Both examine knowledge, neither touches on competency. After passing these examinations all surgeons are assumed to be equally competent in all areas of neurosurgery. It is difficult for one institution to hold out higher standards because this is contrary to our laws. Another major fault is the lack of control over how new procedures are introduced into neurosurgery. Any neurosurgeon can follow any locally approved method to learn a new procedure and bring it to patients. In the history of American neurosurgery there has been only one organized educational effort specifically designed to educate practicing neurosurgeons for the introduction of a new procedure. This was when intradiscal enzyme therapy was legalized and for a short period of time thought to be an important method of therapy for large numbers of patients. Furthermore, our system has no assurance of ongoing competency, outcomes are not assessed in any way.

Thus, the greatest fault of our system is that competency is not ensured. Is this a major issue? I believe it is. In the recent Bosc Report approximately 10% of graduates either questioned their own competence or were questioned by their program directors.

Another issue is that the cost per neurosurgical trainee in the United States now exceeds $100,000 per year without considering the lost income of the trainee. Not only should we re-examine our training programs to ensure that competency can be guaranteed, but we must also be certain that we are using our resources parsimoniously for the training of young neurosurgeons.

No changes of importance have occurred in medical education in the past one hundred years. It is time that we re-examine what we do to address these important issues in medical education.

The Johns Hopkins Competency Program

Any changes which occur must be within the framework of the current requirements of The American Board of Neurological Surgery. Whether competency training will shorten or lengthen the educational program for most residents is immaterial. The important issue is to make sure that the finishing residents are capable of independent practice. It is also important to define what those capabilities are. Therefore, all of our reorganization of training occurs within the framework of current requirements and the changes we make are internal to those requirements. Competency training has three aspects. The first is the acquisition of skills required in neurosurgical practice, the second is the acquisition of knowledge, and the third is the application of that knowledge. They are separate issues and do not occur simultaneously. Skills are the easiest to acquire and, therefore, we begin skills training first.

Year 1

Year 1 is spent in general surgery acquiring basic surgical skills. These include obvious surgical issues such as knot tying, suturing, wound closure and management, and postoperative care. We also include line placement, monitoring and all the issues of intensive care. The trainees in neurosurgery must keep lists of procedures done and their general surgery mentors must assure us that they are competent to do these procedures independently.

Years 2 and 3

Years 2 and 3 are the traditional junior residency years. Residents are now full-time in clinical neursourgery, but we include rotations in neurological intensive care as well. Our residents spend two months in the intensive care unit. We have taken all of the procedures of neurosurgery, listed them in order of increasing complexity, and then divided them into component parts. We have then assigned the sequence in which we would expect the resident to learn to do them. As sequential examples, residents will learn to open and close most incisions during their first year, but will not clip aneurysms until their final year. Some procedures such as lumbar puncture, ventricular tap, or shunt taps are simple and the resident simply keeps lists of procedures done and asks for verification of competency from the staff. Most surgical procedures are complex and broken into component parts. For instance, we have divided laminectomy into: 1) positioning and preparing the patient for surgery, 2) opening the skin and exposing the laminae, 3) closing the wound, and 4) doing the laminectomy. The residents keep lists of participation in each part of the procedure and when they feel themselves competent, they ask for staff verification.

Competency must be verified by two staff members independently and then approved by the program director. Once approved, we believe the resident is competent to carry out that procedure independently, though American law still requires supervision. The point is that the resident is now technically competent to do the procedure and supervision is necessary only to meet the legal requirement. The trainee does not stop doing the procedures when competency is verified. They are expected to continue to add to their list of surgical experience and to improve both speed and technique.

Since all procedures are included in our list, the residents have to participate in all aspects of the program. Our surgical volume is large and includes many very specialized procedures; this requirement ensures that every resident will experience every kind of procedure.

Another advantage in the list keeping is that faculty members understand the obligation to allow residents to participate in surgery and to help them become competent. This surgical experience must always be under the direct supervision of the primary surgeon who is doing the procedure and takes full responsibility for the patient. The residents cannot demand to do anything for which the staff member believes them unprepared. The patient is guaranteed that there is no lapse of quality since all this is accomplished with the resident as first assistant.

As the trainees proceed through the system gaining more and more skills, their duties change. Our experience with this program over the two years of its existence is that junior residents acquire surgical skills much more rapidly than we allowed before. It is my belief that the residents are now at a point in surgical skills at the end of the first year that previously required two years to accomplish. This means that the residents will have the opportunity to move to more specialized areas which can then be infolded into the 36 months of neurosurgery. Examples are the spine service, stereotaxis, endovascular techniques, peripheral

nerve surgery, and pain. The only constant in this two year experience is the call schedule which is necessarily fixed, but the experience during the day may be modified to allow the residents to acquire special skills in a chosen area of interest.

Year 4

Year 4 is the chief residency. Trainees are chief residents on a large pediatric neurosurgery service and chief at an affiliated hospital which has a busy general neurosurgery service. Year 4 completes the 36 months of neurosurgery required.

Years 5 and 6

Years 5 and 6 are usually laboratory years. To become competent independent researchers requires a minimum of two years in my opinion and probably more in many fields. Many of our trainees elect three years or more. A PhD is available to those who wish to pursue the degree and typically takes four to five years. A two year Masters program in clinical research is available throughout our School of Public Health. This is encouraged for those interested in academic practice, but not in basic laboratory research. The goal of this extended laboratory experience is to teach people to do research, not how to think. Scientific method, study design, critical reading, and appropriate use of biostatistics are taught to all in the course of the program and do not require a long laboratory experience to learn in my opinion. Trainees in the clinical research program typically also take special electives in areas of clinical interest. Trainees are allowed to go to other institutions for both research and clinical training. Many come into the program with PhD's and they are encouraged to use the two-year period to begin independent research and to acquire any additional skills that may be useful.

Following the laboratory experience the trainees return for the Halstedian year of supervised practice. They have met all the requirements for the American Board and in two years can sit for the examination. However, we require that the first of these two years be spent in independent practice at Johns Hopkins. During this time they maintain their own clinics, have their own patients, but they still must seek second opinions and operating room assistance. They have the option of continuing to participate in any other specialized surgical procedures with other staff members, particularly vascular disease, spinal instrumentation, and tumor surgery.

In addition to these standard aspects of the program, we have available two-year fellowships which lead to national certification in intensive care and endovascular therapy. Both contain a laboratory experience and are done in lieu of basic research training.

The unique features of this program are all based on the competency issues and enfolding specialized experiences. The competency verification is required and it appears to us that the time generated can be used to expand experience in specialized areas, thus enfolding what might otherwise have been left to a fellowship year after training. This enfolding has no official status and none of these lead to certification, but the added experience is clearly verified.

Acquisition of Knowledge

Skills and knowledge do not track together [5]. In fact there is a considerable body of evidence that indicates that the skills must be obtained first in order for knowledge to be applied efficiently. We have created a parallel case management seminar program which is organized to cover clinical topics in somewhat the same sequence that the skills are being cultivated. These consist of weekly meetings in which patients are presented to the residents emphasizing history and physical examination, diagnostic studies, programs and therapeutic choices, outcomes, and moral and ethical issues. The residents are given a reading list in each topic which is composed of a few of the classic articles. All neurosurgery topics are covered and the course repeats on a two year basis [6].

As a part of the same program, topics entitled, "The Neurosurgeon in Society" are included. These topics include such things as practice management, legal issues, hospital management, organized medicine, and societal medical issues which effect neurosurgeons.

Currently residents also complete a year-long dissection course in surgical anatomy which emphasizes surgical approaches and a laboratory course in microsurgery.

All residents serve as laboratory assistants in the medical school neuroscience course and we are con-

sidering a seminar program in basic science if the case management seminar is successful.

Techniques of Education

Restructuring the program has allowed us to examine educational theory and how people acquire and utilize knowledge. All of our conferences are organized in the mode of adult education. The technical term for this is androgological as opposed to didactic or pedagological which emphasizes the professor as the expert giver of opinion. In the adult educational mode both trainee and staff are students, and both learn together. The trainee takes responsibility for his or her own education, and the staff member serves to inspire, to direct, and to limit fields of study. Those things that can be learned from the literature should be, and the professor provides a synthesis based upon experience which is not available from reading.

The second major issue that must be considered in any resident educational program is the style of learning of the trainees. Some are topic learners and do better when a subject is covered extensively. Some are random learners and will do better with large amounts of material which they synthesize themselves. A third learning style is termed "omnivorous." These individuals generally learn everything without regard to immediate relevance and they need guidance in a field as large as the neurosciences. Subjects have to be presented so that all three groups are served [4].

The fundamental basis of our program is the Rasmussen theory of acquisition and application of knowledge which seems to me to be particularly relevant for neurosurgery. Rasmussen states that one first must learn skills in order to apply knowledge and that these skills are often mastered long before they can be used independently. Then he postulates a rules-based stage in which the trainee has some knowledge, but needs to follow rules that will provide an appropriate answer most of the time. Rules are common in neurosurgery and many neurosurgeons never seem to proceed beyond them. Unfortunately, there are exceptions to all these rules so that following them will produce errors. Nevertheless, following the rules will accurately predict outcome most of the time and is an essential phase. The rules need to be general and not surgeon-based, or the trainees may become lost in a welter of seemingly conflicting opinions when the points of difference are truly trivial [7,8].

Rasmussen's third phase is termed "knowledge-based practice." In this phase the individual has both knowledge and experience and can now individualize to make the best choice rather than following the rule. Knowledge-based practice often appears mysterious to the trainee, and frequently to other physicians who do not have the facility. The rule followers often believe the knowledge-based physician is making capricious decisions or is just lucky. No one knows how to educate any individual to move to the knowledge-based phase, but our program is organized along these principles that allows the opportunity for skills acquisition, learning all the rules, and then individualized choice based upon knowledge and experience [7,8,9].

Verification of Competency

It is obvious that the fundamental issue is the assurance of competency. If this kind of program is to be successful, it is necessary to have an adequate clinical volume to allow its implementation. In each of the clinical years, each resident can participate in about 400 operations each. During the year of supervised practice, the trainee can choose from over 1,000 procedures each, and typically is involved in more than 400 operations during that year. Any systemic deficiencies in the program become immediately apparent when these kinds of records are kept.

The second issue is length of training. It is my view that we are beyond the time when fixed periods of training are required. We should concentrate on the acquisition of skills and verifying competency. While times are still fixed by the Board, I can envision an era in which there is no specified time of training and all training is based upon demonstrated competency. Whether this will require more or less time than our current standards is uncertain. Training time can be saved by enfolding specialty training thus avoiding the increasing number of fellowship years for special experiences. Reducing time reduces cost.

Another very costly aspect of current training is obligatory laboratory time for those who will never become independent researchers or continue a laboratory interest. The cost is great and another trainee may be deprived of a position in the neurosciences. I believe research training should be equally tailored to the aspirations and talents of the individual

trainee. A small number will become serious competitive basic researchers and they should be given the opportunity to acquire and use these skills in residency training. A larger group will apply basic techniques to neurosurgical programs and they need to be encouraged. There is a great need for well-trained clinical researchers and this should be an option. Everyone needs to learn scientific method, critical thinking, appropriate use of statistics, and what constitutes good study design. These can easily be taught and the trainee does not need extensive laboratory time to learn these principles. There is good evidence that individuals do not transfer general principles from one field to another so it is better that these concepts be taught in the context in which they will be used in practice.

The residency program developed by Halsted remains one of the great educational achievements. The rise of modern medicine is due in major part to this concept of organized postgraduate education in specific fields. Even when expanded by a defined competency verification, the process stops at the end of training. In our current system surgeons who have completed training and passed all the requisite Board examinations are considered to be equals with no differentiation in skills. There is no ongoing verification of competency. Nothing ensures that the surgeon stays current. Only outcome studies are likely to do this, reexamination cannot. Another fault is in the introduction of new procedures. There is no specified way in which any physician learns to apply a new procedure. We need to codify what is required to master a new procedure and use it with patients. A program of this kind should not be restrictive. That is, all qualified surgeons should be able to use new procedures for their patients, but the way in which the new skill is learned and applied needs to be specified and not left up to the individual or hospital. Postgraduate medical education opportunities are many and varied. Most neurosurgeons are very conscientious about meeting attendance. The issue is not knowledge, but rather the acquisition of a new skill.

It has been 100 years since the residency system of postgraduate medical education was introduced. My suggestions are not fundamental changes. The concept is as valid at the end of the century as it was at the beginning. Rather they are embellishments to ensure competency and practice-long learning. In addition, a profession is defined by its ability to regulate itself. The concept of lifelong learning needs to incorporate outcome assessment to both guarantee the public the best medical care and to guide the learning process.

The Selection Process

There are two other issues in the American system that require comment. Both are included in the selection process. Students usually choose a specialty in their junior year and are matched to that specialty midway through their senior year. Ten percent of those who choose neurosurgery find they have made the wrong career choice and change to another field of medicine. There is no harm in this, but it is wasteful of both time and money. Another 10% are found to be unsuitable for neurosurgery and are discharged by their program directors. This is good for it protects the public, but does indicate there is a need for improving the selection process. The data indicate that discharge usually occurs because the trainee is found to be psychologically ill matched to neursourgery.

Competency remains the most important issue. The fact that some trainees were concerned about the quality of their training reflects upon the training programs. That some program directors were concerned about the competency of those completing their programs may indicate a problem in the trainee or the program or both. This group of physicians is most concerning because they will be practicing neurosurgeons. If competency is verified throughout training, we will have no concerns about the surgical and patient management skills of the individuals who finish our programs. The verification of competency also forces a close look at the experience available in all training programs and separates exposure from experience for the trainees. If programs are found wanting the requisite number of cases, either those programs will have to lose the privilege of training residents or ways will have to be found to ensure the residents obtain necessary experience through rotations in other programs.

The Goal

The motto of the Johns Hopkins Department of Neurosurgery is "Teknae, Epistame, Pathos." The Greeks, as usual, had very appropriate words to describe our desired attributes. Teknae means "manual skill raised to the level of beauty," Epistame means "knowledge of unusual depth and breadth," and Pathos means "an unquenchable desire to know the unknown." All we really have to do in training is be sure that these three characteristics continue to define all neurosurgeons.

References

1. Muller S (1986) The post Gutenberg University. Johns Hopkins APL Technical Digest 7(1):108–112
2. Muller S (1985) Wilhelm von Humboldt and The University in the United States. Johns Hopkins APL Technical Digest 6(3):253–256
3. Eliot CW (1893) Report of the Committee of Ten on Secondary School Studies. Government Printing Office, Washington DC
4. Long DM (1996) Editorial. Educating neurosurgeons for the 21st century. Neurosurg Quart 6(2):78–88
5. Blum BI, Sigilliot VG (1986) An expert system for designing information systems. Johns Hopkins APL Technical Digest 7(1):23–31
6. Rasmussen J (1983) Skills, rules, knowledge: signals, signs and symbols and other distinctions in human performance models. IEEE Trans Systems, Man and Cybernetics 123:257–66
7. Rasmussen J, Lind M (1982) A model of human decision making in complex systems and its use for design of system control strategies. Riso National Laboratory Report. Riso-M-2349, Roskilde, Denmark
8. Larkin JH (1977) Skilled problem solving in experts. Technical Report in Science and Mathematics Education. University of California, Berkeley
9. Tamblyn RM, Klass DJ, Schnabl GK, Kopelow ML (1991) The accuracy of standardized-patient presentations. Med Educ 25:100–109

Correspondence: Prof. D. M. Long, M.D., Ph.D., Department of Neurosurgery, Johns Hopkins University School of Medicine, Meyer 7-109, 600 North Wolfe Street, Baltimore, Maryland 21287-7709, U.S.A.

Acta Neurochir (1997) [Suppl] 69:65–69
© Springer-Verlag 1997

The UEMS Model – Proposals for Classification and Training Durations of Specialties Registered in Doctors' Directives

L. Calliauw

Chief Editor, Acta Neurochirurgica, Brussels, Belgium

Keywords: UEMS model, training duration, training contents.

Introduction

Founded in 1958, less than one year after the treaty of Rome, the European Union of Medical Specialists (UEMS) groups together specialist doctors regardless of their field or mode of practice, or their legal status. Its object is the advancement and harmonisation of the quality of specialist medical practice in Europe and the defence, at international level, of the status of the medical specialist and of his/her professional role in society (Table 1).

The UEMS, in cooperation with the Standing Committee of European Doctors (CP), participated in the drafting of the European Directives governing the free movement of doctors and mutual recognition of medical credentials throughout the European Community which were adopted by the Council of the European Community in 1975 and came into effect in 1976.

UEMS played a major role in the elaboration of the reports and recommendations issued by the Advisory Committee on Medical Training (ACMT) on April 5th 1979, March 11th 1981, March 9th 1983 and June 20th 1985. These various reports to a very large extent reflect UEMS views on the training of specialist doctors and the practice of specialised medicine.

The Policy of UEMS

1. The Definition of Specialist Medicine

The specialist doctor has chosen to confine his or her practice essentially to one field of medicine. This implies that he or she shall be, and must remain, at a high level of competence in the chosen specialty by mastering advances and innovations both in data and technique.

For some specialties the expansion of knowledge threatens to lead to super-specialties concentrating on particular techniques or a narrowly defined field of pathology. National authorities often grant official recognition to these competences, which should however remain within the broad framework of the main specialty. These developments should not lead to the proliferation of new specialties, as the number of specialties must be kept under control. The development of techniques should not prevent awareness that specialised medicine is a clinical discipline which must remain focussed upon the patient.

Clearly the practice of the general practitioner and the medical specialist are complementary. Their precise roles and arrangements for access to specialist treatment vary from country to country. Patients should be able to exercise freedom of choice, and should have prompt access to the treatment which they need, within the framework of the health care system of the country in which they live. Good practice in both disciplines depends on effective cooperation and exchange of information.

2. Medical Specialist Training

a) The Competent Body

At national level, the training of medical specialists is regulated by a National Authority, which may be a

Table 1. *Composition and Functioning of U.E.M.S.*

The UEMS was founded in 1958 with the aim of defending, at international lever, the status of the medical specialist and his professional role in society. Its membership is composed of the national medical association representing medical specialists in each of its member countries, at the rate of one per country. At present it includes 17 full members:

– Germany	Gemeinschaft Fachärztlicher Berufsverbände
– Austria	Österreichische Ärztekammer
– Belgium	Groupement des Unions Prof. Belges de Médecins Spécialistes
– Denmark	Danish Medical Association
– Spain	Consejo General de Colegios Oficiales de Médicos
– Finland	Finnish Medical Association
– France	Union Nationale des Médecins Spécialistes Confédérés
– Greece	Panhellenic Medical Association
– Ireland	The Irish Medical Organisation
– Italy	Federazione Nazionale degli Ordini dei Medici
– Luxembourg	Association des Médecins et Médecins-Dentistes du Grand-Duché de Luxembourg
– Norway	Norwegian Medical Association
– The Netherlands	Landelijke Specialisten Vereniging
– Portugal	Ordem dos Medicos
– U. Kingdom	British Medical Association
– Sweden	Swedish Medical Association
– Switzerland	Fédération des Médecins Suisses

i.e. the countries of the European Union and Norway and Switzerland.

Associate members are Hungary (Federation of Hungarian Medical Societies, Motesz), Malta (The Medical Association of Malta), Slovenia (Zdravniska Zbornica Sloveije) and Turkey (Turkish Medical Association).

The *Management Council* is composed of two delegates from each country, who represent their country rather than their specialty. Since its foundation, the principle of one vote per country has been observed. Each delegation may be strengthened by one or more experts. Associate members sit in an advisory capacity.

At least two plenary assemblies are held each year

combination of competent professional or University bodies, a National Board or a national governmental authority receiving advice from professional organisations. It sets standards in accordance with national rules and EU legislation as well as considering UEMS recommendations for recognition of training programmes, of trainers and training centres, the quality assurance of training, the qualifications of the medical specialist and manpower planning.

b) Guarantee of the Quality of Training

– Basic medical training should be authenticated before the course of specialist training is started. The specialist training must be comprehensive and should omit no important field.
– In the training centers, adequate numbers of teaching staff and appropriate training facilities must be available and in balance with the number of trainees in order to guarantee high quality training.
– Other methods of ensuring the quality of training could include, for example, the audit, logbook, the possibility of part of the training period being spent abroad, and a national examination at the end of the postgraduate training.

c) Particular Aspects of Specialist Training

The content and practice of the specialty inevitably determine the training that is required. A system of centralised classification which takes into account the real content of each specialty and its historical development shows that training in medical and surgical specialties follows different pathways. However, apart from these main groupings, there exist organ-related disciplines which include both medical and surgical elements.

This type of classification allows one to define a specialist training programme based on a common trunk, which broadens out to include the divisions and subdivisions of both medical and surgical specialties.

A regrouping of specialties such as was proposed in 1983 by the Advisory Committee on Medical Training (ACMT) should adopted in place of the classification in Articles 26 and 27 of the existing Medical Directives, which take no account of the relationship of the specialties to one another (see Appendix 1).

As regards the content of training and the relation of the Common Trunk to specialist training, the work of the UEMS Sections and European Boards has resulted in the publication, in October 1995, of a more accurate definition. At the same time, a precise definition of the content of training should not be taken to imply that specialist practice is a system of watertight compartments. Because disciplines frequently overlap, there must be scope for flexibility, although quite clearly no specialist should carry out a procedure for which he or she is not appropriately trained.

3. Continuing Medical Education (CME)

Continuing medical education is both a necessity and an obligation, which applies as much to the medical profession as to any other. The process of education lasts throughout the doctor's entire career, beginning with basic undergraduate training, carrying on through specialist training and extending for the remainder of professional life as Continuing Medical Education.

As it is a professional, ethical and moral obligation, CME must be managed and supervised independently by the profession.

Basically, it should be a voluntary responsibility for the individual specialist. The representative national professional organisation is free to decide in a democratic manner to impose a formal obligation to fulfil CME requirements. However, someone who does not fulfil these requirements cannot lose his/her status as a doctor or specialist, but must understand that he/she may be disadvantaged in other ways.

The content of CME must take into account the specific situation of the specialist and in consequence is of an individual nature. Systems of assessment which award credit points are preferable to those which involve re-evaluation or recertification of the specialist's knowledge. Control of such systems must remain in the hands of organisations which represent the medical community. These systems could also include models of self-assessment.

4. The Organisation of Specialist Medicine

The activity of the specialist doctor may be practised not only in a hospital or private office, but also in health centres, companies, schools and other places where the specialist's presence is required. In all cases the specialist doctor shall be free to treat his/her patient without external constraint.

The medical specialist must have adequate medical equipment at his/her disposal. The quality of care should remain independent from the system of remuneration, and compliance with professional quality standards should be assured by Peer Review assessment.

Contracts with and the remuneration of specialists, whether salaried or in private practice, must provide for the expenses involved for the doctor in meeting his/her CME obligations.

Independence from outside pressure in the choice of management and treatment of the individual patient remains the cornerstone of medical care. The physician and the patient must remain free to exercise a responsible choice.

Conclusions

The UEMS, through its 34 Specialist Sections,* is in a position to know the conditions which each specialty needs to meet in order to reach harmonisation, both as regards the duration and the content of training and the practice of the various disciplines registered in the Medical Directives. It can inform each EU member state of these conditions, in all countries and all specialties.

Thanks to the European Boards, which are the working groups of the Specialist Sections, and include delegates appointed by scientific and academic bodies as well as representatives of the Sections, the UEMS is in a position to define for each discipline the conditions which will ensure high quality training and the necessary criteria for a training centre. It can put forward suggestions regarding methods of assessment to which individuals can submit if they so desire.

---

* The *Specialist Sections* were created in 1962 and are composed of experts in each discipline. At present, there are 34 specialist sections representing 43 of the 50 specialties registered in the EU Medical Directives. Consisting of two delegates per country, the sections lead an independent existence. They report to the Management Council, which co-ordinates their activities.

Since 1990, each section has been empowered to establish a European Board for its specialty with the appointment of delegates from the scientific and academic sectors. These are in reality working groups whose main objective is to guarantee the highest standards of care in the field of the specialty concerned in the countries of the EU by ensuring that the medical specialist training is raised to the highest possible level.

The UEMS collaborates actively with the Standing Committee of European Doctors where it is represented by a Liaison Officer.

UEMS maintains continuing relations with other European medical organisations such as the European Union of General Practitioners (UEMO), the European Academy for Medical Training (EAMF), the Permanent Working Group of Junior Hospital Doctors (PWG), the European Association of Hospital Doctors (AEMH) and the European Association of Salaried Doctors (FEMS).

It also maintains close contact with the authorities of the European Union and the Council of Europe

Appendix 1: Proposals for Classification and Training Durations of the Specialties Registered in the Doctor's Directives

These proposals take into account the conclusions of the report published by the Advisory Committee on Medical Training in 1983, and the evolution of the situation of the specialties in the different countries.

1. Group of the Medical Specialties
   a) *Adult internal medecine*: 6-year training experience in one or more medical specialties
      Medical specialties requiring a strong experience in internal medicine: 6-year training
      2-year common trunk in internal medicine, 3 years achieved in clinical practice in the specialty concerned, 1 year may be devoted to research or to training in a closely related discipline.
      – cardiology*
      – endocrinology*
      – gastro-enterology*
      – general haematology*
      – renal diseases*
      – respiratory medicine*
      – rheumatology*
   b) *Child and Adolescent internal medicine (paediatrics)*: 5-year training
      Medical specialties requiring a strong experience in paediatrics: 5-year training
      3-year commun trunk in paediatrics, 2 years achieved in clinical practice in the specialty concerned
      – cardiology*
      – endocrinology*
      – gastro-enterology*
      – general hematology*
      – renal diseases*
      – respiratory medicine*
      – rheumatology*
      Allergology: 5-year training with a common trunk in internal medicine
      Neurology: 6-year training, including 4 years in neurology*,**
      Dermato-Venereology

Dermatology   4-year training
Venereology
Tropical medicine
Geriatrics   4-year training
Infectious diseases
with common trunk in internal medicine

2. Group of Surgical Specialties
   General surgery: *6-year* training
   Common trunk with the other surgical specialties
   Surgical specialties requiring a training of 6 years with common trunk in surgery
   – orthopaedic surgery
   – urology
   – plastic surgery
   – thoracic surgery
   – paediatric surgery
   – vascular surgery
   – gastro-enterological surgery
   Surgical specialties requiring an experience in parent specialties, and cephalic specialties:
   – neurosurgery: *6-year training*, out of which two years in parent disciplines, including basic neurological sciences
   – oto-rhino-laryngology: *6-year* training*
   – maxillo-facial surgery (basic medical training): *6-year* training including a strong training in stomatology
   – oro-maxillo-facial surgery (basic medical training and of dental art practitioner): *6-year* training, out of which two may be dedicated to the award of the legal diploma in odontology
   – ophthalmology: *4-year* training
   – stomatology: *4-year* training

3. Mixt Group
   Anaesthesiology-reanimation: 5-year training
   Physical and rehabilitation medicine: 5-year training
   Radiations medicine: common trunk in radiological theory
   – radiodiagnosis: *5-years*
   – radiotherapy: *5-years*
   – radiology (combined): *6-years*
   Nuclear medicine: *4-year* training

4. Obstetrics-gynaecology: *5-year training*, with common truck for the different sub-specialties.

5. Laboratory Medicine
   a) *5-year* training
      – pathological anatomy

---

* a possible period of transition should be foreseen.
** for paediatric neurology, a 3-year common trunk in paediatrics should be foreseen

---

* a possible transition period should be foreseen

b) *5-year* training with clinical experience (1 year of common trunk in internal medicine):
  - medical biopathology (clinical biology)
  - biological haematology
  - microbiology
  - biological chemistry
  - immunology

6. Psychiatry

5-year including a common trunk in neurology
  - psychiatry
  - child and adolescent psychiatry

6-year training including a common trunk in neurology
  - neuro-psychiatry

7. Miscellaneous
  - "Community medicine" (public health): *4-year* training
  - pharmacology: *4-year* training
  - occupational medicine: *4-year* training

Publications

Documents available at the U.E.M.S. secretariat, 20, avenue de la Couronne, B-1050 Brussels, Belgium.

Advisory Committee on Medical Training

- Reports, opinions and recommendations adopted by the Commission during the first term of office of its members (from 6 April 1976 to 5 April 1970), published on January 3d 1980.
- Opinion on the mutual recognition of training periods completed in another member state as part of specialist training, published on March 11, 1981.
- Second report recommendations on the training of specialists adopted by the Committee at its meeting on 8 and 9 March 1983.
- Third report and recommendations on the conditions for specialist training adopted by the committee at its meeting on 18 and 20 June 1985, published on March 4th 1986.

European Union of Medical Specialists

- Compendium of Medical Specialist Training in the E.C. (December 1992)
- Minutes of the meeting of the representatives of the U.E.M.S. Monospecialist Sections (D 9157) – European Boards
- Minutes of the meeting of representatives of Laboratory Medicine (D 9264)
- Minutes of the meeting of the representatives of the UEMS Monospecialist Sections (D 9221) – training durations
- Study of the training durations for the Medical Specialists in the E.C. (D 9248)
- Motion of the U.E.M.S. Monospecialist Sections concerning the adaptation of the training durations in the Doctors' Directives (D 9339)
- U.E.M.S. proposals on the adaptation of the E.C. Medical Directives (CP 93/105)
- Motion concerning the number of specialties (D 9327)
- Minutes of the meeting of the representatives of Internal Pathology (D 9332)
- Motion concerning harmonisation of training in Internal Medicine and allied specialties within the E.C. (D 9330)
- Minutes of the meeting of the representatives of the UEMS Monospecialist Sections (D 9342)
- Charter on training of medical specialists in the European Community (D 9367 bis)
- Minutes of the meeting of the representatives of the UEMS Specialist Sections (D 9456) – Continuing Medical Education (CME)
- Charter on continuing medical education of medical specialists in the European Union (D 9426 bis)
- The position of the U.E.M.S. in regard to the Continuing Medical Education (CME) of specialists (D 9451)
- Autonomy of specialist medical practice (D 9467)
- European Training Charter for medical specialists (1995)

Correspondence: Prof. L. Calliauw, Office Acta Neurochirurgica, Kroonlaan 20, B-1050 Brussels, Belgium

Acta Neurochir (1997) [Suppl] 69:70–72
© Springer-Verlag 1997

Contents and Structure of a Training Program. The Japanese Proposal

T. Yoshimoto and **T. Tominaga**

Tohoku University School of Medicine, Sendai, Japan

Keywords: Training program, Japan, contents, structure.

Medical System in Japan

It is not easy to standardize training programs for neurosurgery, because it should respond to the demands of each area or country. Do you know which nation has the highest average life expectancy in the world? The current average life expectancy of the Japanese is the highest in the world! In my view, an integrated medical insurance system and local medical care systems are particularly important for expansion of life expectancy in Japan. None of the citizens miss medical service when they become sick in Japan, because all Japanese people have medical insurance supported by the government. On the other hand, Japanese people desire to receive medical care through a local medical system, staying in their family, and do not necessarily want to receive medical care through famous doctors or institutes. This is unique, as compared with the tendency seen in the Western countries. This is also true for patients who need neurosurgical treatment.

In Japan, the job of a neurosurgeon is not doing operations only. For instance, a typical Japanese neurosurgeon has to manage a patient with subarachnoid hemorrhage as follows: preparation of acceptance at the hospital, examinations including angiography, diagnosis, acute-phase management to prevent re-rupture, and operation. After the operation, he also takes care to prevent vasospasm and manages the general care approximately for one month in the hospital and, afterwards, as an out-patient to support return to work. Japanese neurosurgeons must achieve all those managements for each patient with consistency.

Next, I would like to present the current neurosurgical service in Miyagi-prefecture which government is located at Sendai. Miyagi prefecture consists of 2.3-million population, and has 16 emergency hospitals with a neurosurgical department. Eighty doctors are in the service in the neurosurgical departments in this area. Half of them are residents and the other half are neurosurgeons authorized by the Japanese board. However, in my opinion, 20 more doctors would be required for an ideal service in this area.

Residency Training System

The Japanese Neurosurgical Board [1]

The residency training protocol is based on the requirements of the neurosurgical board, which is controlled by the Japan Neurosurgical Society. This protocol has been in force since 1966, and is assumed to be an important and essential system to elevate the standard of clinical practice and neurosurgical science in Japan. In this system, a candidate for the board must have been trained for 6 or more years in one of the hospitals authorized by the Japan Neurosurgical Society. In this period, a candidate has to study in neurosurgical clinics for at least 3 years, and is usually engaged in neuroscience research for rest of this period. A candidate for the board must present an operation list recording 100 cases done by himself, including 20 cases of brain tumors, 20 cases of either cerebral aneurysms or AVMs, and 20 cases of either pediatric, traumatic, functional, or spinal surgery.

Every 2 years, all neurosurgeons vote to elect the examiners of the board examination. The test consists of a written and an oral examination prepared by the examiners. The written examination includes 250 questions, 40 of them on neuroscience, 70 on brain tumor and infection, 70 on vascular and functional neurosurgery, and 70 on pediatric, traumatic, and spinal neurosurgery. The oral examination consists of three parts: brain tumor and infection, vascular disease and functional neurosurgery, and pediatric, traumatic, and spinal surgery. They focus on operative procedures and post-operative management. Usually, almost 60% of the applicants pass the board.

Contents of Residency Training (Table 1)

During the first two years of a six-year program, they learn general patient care, neurology, neuroradiology, and emergency care. Thereafter, they are engaged for two years in neuroscience research and subspecialties, such as endovascular surgery and stereotactic radiosurgery. They will apply for the board examination following the last two years of training, where they perform major operations and perioperative patient management.

The technical training in the first and second year is as follows: (1) spinal tap, (2) intubation and extubation, (3) tracheostomy, (4) cerebral angiography, (5) burr hole, (6) V-P shunt, (7) depressed fracture, (8) skull tumor, (9) chronic subdural hematoma, (10) cranioplasty, and (11) craniotomy.

The technical training for the third and fourth year is as follows: (1) acute epidural hematoma, (2) acute subdural hematoma, (3) subfrontal exploration, (4) superficial solitary brain tumor, (5) intercerebral hematoma, (6) opening of Sylvian fissure, (7) carotid artery ligation, (8) spinal laminectomy.

In the two years, residents receive the following technical training: (1) meningocele, (2) encephalocele, (3) craniosynostosis, (4) convexity meningioma, (5) sphenoid wing meningioma, (6) posterior fossa tumor, (7) neurovascular decompression, (8) endarterectomy, (9) pituitary adenoma (transsphenoid), (10) STA-MCA anastomosis, (11) IC-PC aneurysm, (12) MCA aneurysm, (13) AVM.

University Hospital and Affiliated Hospital

The university hospital has to achieve its own clinical service, basic research, and education for medical students. At the same time, the university hospital also has to play an important role to organize the affiliated training hospitals to function well (Fig. 1). The organization of the university hospital and the affiliated hospitals renders it possible to conduct clinical studies, such as stroke patient-, brain tumor patient-, and head trauma patient-registry projects. The stroke patient-registry indicates that one out of 1000 citizen of Miyagi prefecture is hospitalized per year in a neurosurgical department for the treatment of stroke.

The neurosurgical department of the Tohoku University has eight full-time neurosurgeons; one chairman who is responsible for general management and one associate professor specialized in vascular and cranial base surgery. The other six are appointed as assistant professors, specialized in either pediatric neurosurgery, pituitary surgery, spinal surgery, stereotactic surgery, magnetic encephalography, and malignant brain tumor. We can not provide all training programs with the university hospital alone. Therefore, it is particularly important for the resi-

Table 1. *Residency Training*

Year	Contents	Operations
1st	general patient care neurology, neuroradiology	ventricular drainage chronic subdural hematoma
2nd	emergency care etc.	V-P shunt, skull tumor, etc.
3rd	neuroscience research endovascular surgery	intracerebral hematoma acute epidural hematoma
4th	stereotactic surgery etc.	spinal laminectomy, etc.
5th	major operations perioperative mangement	aneurysm (IC-PC, etc.), AVM convexity meningioma
6th		posterior fossa tumor etc.
7th	the Japanese Board of Neurological Surgery	

MIYAGI prefecture

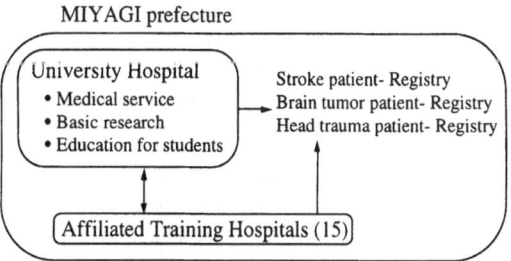

Fig. 1

dents to be trained at the affiliated hospitals. The residents attend several affiliated hospitals during the 6 years of their training period. So cooperation between the university hospital and the affiliated hospitals is essential to the Japanese style of residency training. One of the most important jobs of the chairman is to equally rotate the residents to the affiliated hospitals.

In total 45 residents have joined our department; from 1990 to 1994 nine residents per year on average. The School of medicine in our university consists of 25 clinical and 30 basic research departments. Approximately 100 students graduate per year, and they usually join a certain department of alma mater. Therefore, the number of residents joining the neurosurgical department seems quite high. Eight doctors, 18% of our residents, had previously been trained in general surgical departments, and four doctors, 9% of our residents, dropped out of our department.

Neuroscience Research

Neuroscience research during the six-year training period is very significant. The staff members of the university hospital supervise neuroscience research of the residents, sometimes in collaboration with a basic research department. The goal of the research is to obtain a Ph.D. degree from our medical school. The research period principally depends on the contents of research. Residents can apply for a Ph.D. immediately after completion of the residency train-

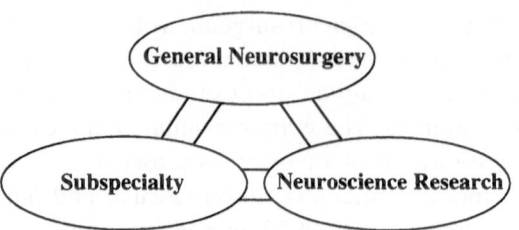

Fig. 2. Structure of Neurosurgical Training

ing; thus the minimum period required for a Ph.D. is seven years. Table 2 shows the research groups in my department and their current research projects. In Japan, a neurosurgeon is evaluated by his achievements in neuroscience research, as well as by his surgery. Research can also be conducted abroad, i.e. in research laboratories all over the world. For example, eight out of 41 residents in our department have conducted their studies in the United States. Another important job of the chairman is to manage neuroscience research properly.

An Ideal Structure of Neurosurgical Training (Fig. 2)

I would like to address the importance of two further subspecialties, endovascular surgery and stereotactic radiosurgery. These two modalities should be performed by neurosurgeons and their integration within our speciality is important. In other words, neurosurgeons must address not only surgical operations, but also these modalities to care for patients more comprehensively. In addition, fundamental neuroscience research can support general neurosurgery as well as the subspecialties. Neurosurgery as a speciality in Japan has tremendously developed during the past 50 years only with the support and cooperation of Western countries. I strongly believe that the future of neurosurgery depends essentially on the unity of these three areas – general neurosurgery and our speciality will achieve even greater success, if these three areas work in harmony.

References

1. Kikuchi H (1995) Post-graduate education of neurosurgeons in Japan. Neurosurgeons 14:9–18 (English Abstract)

Correspondence: Prof. T. Yoshimoto, M.D., Ph.D., Department of Neurosurgery, Tohoku University School of Medicine, 1-1 Seiryo-machi, Aoba-ku, Sendai 980-77, Japan

Table 2. *Neuroscience Research*

Groups	Current Reseach Projects
– Brain tumors	genomic analysis of glioma
– Pituitary tumors	TGF-β receptors, cell cycle related proteins
– Pediatric neurosurgery	anaerobic metabolism in hydrocephalus
– Brain ischemia	growth factor receptors, nitric oxide
– Brain trauma	wound healing, vasospasm
– Intravascular therapy	LASER therapy for atherosclerosis
– MR spectroscopy	functional imaging
– MEG	functional mapping
– Functional neurosurgery	γ-knife for kindling rat
– Spinal surgery	biomechanics of cervical instrumentations

Acta Neurochir (1997) [Suppl] 69:73–74

Neurosurgical Training in Austria – Present Status and Aspects for the Future

G. Pendl

Department of Neurosurgery, Karl-Franzens University, Graz, Austria

Keywords: Neurosurgical training, Austria.

The Present

Neurosurgical training in Austria is characterized by individual concepts of the 3 medical school departments as well as 6 departments at community hospitals. Thus, the situation in Austria is comparable with many European countries [2]. In addition in Austria, neurosurgery as an individual and distinct speciality evolved at the various sites at different times with different background.

Neurosurgery until 1974 was a speciality within general surgery and the training had to comply with criteria of general surgery with all its aspects and requirements. The first neurosurgical unit was established during World War II in an airforce hospital in Bad Ischl in the Austrian Alps (in 1969 it was moved to the neurological-psychiatric hospital in Linz); in 1963 the Department of Neurosurgery was established at the University of Graz, in 1964 at the University Medical School in Vienna and in 1979 at the University of Innsbruck. Since then further community hospital departments were established in Salzburg, Vienna, Klagenfurt, Dornbirn as well as in Krems. However, it was not before 1974 that Neurosurgery became an independent and distinct speciality of medicine.

The present training program consists of

- five years clinical neurosurgical training
- six months training in general surgery (optional three months of either orthopedics, vascular surgery or traumatology)
- six months training in neurology (optional three months training in neuropathology)

After completion of training as a specialist in neurosurgery, an additional three-year training period in neurological/neurosurgical intensive care medicine as an addititional speciality may be added [5].

The neurosurgical log book requires:

- surgery ("Eingriffe") of tumourous, infectious and vascular diseases of the brain, skull, spine and medulla
- trauma surgery of the skull, brain, medulla and spine
- surgery for pain, birth defects of the brain and medulla
- surgery of peripheral nerves and autonomous nerve system
- knowledge of intracranial stereotactic brain surgery

So far no definite number of any of these specific surgical procedures has been established. A proposed amendment ("Ärztegesetznovelle") in July 1996 for the upcoming year 1997 demands a board examination for any specialist in medicine at the end of training. Specification of those amendments are vague [3].

The Austrian Neurosurgical Society and its individual members are aware that legal pressure imposed by the Austrian Medical Association, political as well as bureaucratic influences are not supporting the aim of the future training with all its aspects of recruitment, selection and conduct. A flow sheet and log book with the documentation of various diagnostic and surgical procedures among other requisites might replace a board examination [1,4,6].

The Future

There is a need to organize and standardize neurosurgical training in Europe. In this context, the results of a questionnaire concerning the future of neurosurgical training and board examinations in Austria are of interest. This questionnaire was distributed among the members of the Austrian Neurosurgical Society in 1996. The questions had a future oriented basis with regard to the European community and its implications. It was not aimed to establish a specific concept of neurosurgical training. The following results were obtained.

Questionnaire and Results

1. Should the residency be modeled according to
   a) Austrian criteria   9%
   b) European Union   82%
   c) others?   9%
2. Quantity of residents
   a) restricted by a federal agency   26%
   b) individually chosen by the states   66%
   c) others   8%
3. Requirements to be fulfilled by future residents
   a) general basis   54%
   b) additional specifics   46%
   (neurological/surgical experience 16, internship 4, military service 3, scientific interest 3)
4. Selection of residents by
   a) a central agency   4%
   b) the hospitals   96%
5. Length of residency
   a) status quo   93%
   b) shortened   0%
   c) lengthened   7%
6. EU working hour regulation – what is the impact on education?
   a) positive   14%
   b) negative   56%
   c) none   30%

7. Board examination
   a) none   11%
   b) at the end of residency   79%
   c) 2 years after residency   10%
8. Board examination – what is a suitable language?
   a) German   56%
   b) English   18%
   c) both   26%
9. Board examination – what is the favorite method?
   a) written   26%
   b) oral   20%
   c) both   54%
10. The importance of training in special areas of neurosurgery was answered as follows:

Neurotraumatology	45	80%
Spine surgery	41	73%
Neurointensive medicine	34	61%
Peripheral nerve surgery	26	46%
Cerebrovascular surgery including AVM	25	45%
Pediatric neurosurgery	20	36%
Functional neurosurgery	16	29%
Endoscopy	11	20%
Radiosurgery	7	13%
Extracranial vascular surgery	7	13%

References

1. Barolin GS, Stellamor K (1996) Das "Rasterzeugnis": eine wichtige Chance zur Qualitätssicherung und Verbesserung der Ärzte-Aus-, Fort- und Weiterbildung in Österreich. ÖKZ 37:50–57
2. Brock M (1996) Neurosurgical training across Europe. In: Palmer JD (ed) Neurosurgery 96. Manual of neurosurgery. Churchill Livingstone, New York, pp 5–6
3. Bundesgesetzblatt für die Republik Österreich 378. Bundesgesetz: Änderung des Ärztegesetzes 1984 und Ausbildungsvorbehaltsgesetz (NR: GP XX RV 150 AB 203 S. 32. BR: AB 5209 S 615.) 31. Juli 1996, 123. Stück, Wien
4. Feil W (1996) Facharztausbildung – Die Praktiker bestimmen, wo es lang geht. BÖC aktuell 4:3–6
5. Schwamberger H (1995) Ärztegesetz 1984 (Stand 1.1. 1995) mit Verordnungen, Erläuterungen und Verweisen. Verlag Österreich, Edition Juristische Literatur, Wien
6. Waclawiczek HW (1995) Aus dem Fortbildungsreferat der Österreichischen Gesellschaft für Chirurgie. Tradition-Gegenwart-Zukunft. Mitt d Öst Ges f Chir 42:13–16

Correspondence: Prof. Dr. G. Pendl, Universitätsklinik für Neurochirurgie, Auenbruggerplatz 29, A-8036 Graz, Austria

Acta Neurochir (1997) [Suppl] 69:75–78

A Resident's Experience and Suggestion

J. Cabiol

Department of Neurosurgery, Ciutat Sanitaria I, Universitaria de Bellvitge, University of Barcelona, Barcelona, Spain

Keywords: Resident experience, resident suggestion.

Introduction

I finished my residency in neurosurgery in December 1995 at the Hospital de Bellvitge of the University of Barcelona. Since the beginning of this year I am a member of the staff of the neurosurgical department at the same institution. I would like to present some thoughts from the other side of the fence, the side of the trainee.

"Der Singer Meisterschlag gewinnt sich nicht an einem Tag." [1]
Richard Wagner. Die Meistersinger von Nürnberg

The first performance of "Die Meistersinger" took place in Munich in June 1868. This magnificent opera is plenty of suggestions about the training process, and Wagner was correct when he said that learning requires more than one day.

Personal Experiences

Let me begin by reporting about my training in neurosurgery. I finished medical school in 1989. I participated in the Spanish National exam for access to training medical specialities in 1990 and I was fortunate enough to obtain a good qualification to apply for training in neurosurgery. In that year there were only 6 new resident positions in neurosurgery in Spain and there were appliants from 32 hospitals. My first choice for a residency was the Hospital de Bellvitge of the University of Barcelona, and I was accepted. The Hospital de Bellvitge is a 950 bed university hospital (level 3) with a fully equipped neurosurgical department, headed by Professor Isamat. The department has 48 beds in the wards, an intermediate care unit of 4 beds and an intensive care unit outside, but intimately related to the department. Two operating rooms with advanced technology for scheduled cases and a third operating room in the casualty department allow an average number of 1,000 surgical procedures per year. There is no paediatric neurosurgery, that means patients of less than 14 years. The neurosurgical department supplies an area of 2.000.000 inhabitants. The team is composed of eight certified neurosurgeons, three residents and one foreign fellow.

My training in neurosurgery spanned over the years 1991 to 1995. My first year was a rotation through related disciplines (general surgery, plastic surgery, neuroradiology, intensive care unit, neurology, and the emergency department). For the remaining four years, I was introduced in a program of progressive responsibility and involvement, both at the ward and in the OR. I had rotations with the different groups in the department, in neurooncology, neurotraumatology, vascular surgery, pituitary tumors, skull base and radiosurgery. New technical developments, such as endoscopic and endovascular procedures, were also available and I participated actively when my patients needed these techniques. I have been satisfied with the idea of progressive responsibility. During my 5th year, I organized my own outpatient clinic and my own surgical acticvity. I had to make my own decisions at the ward and in the OR. My cases were discussed in clinical rounds with the remaining staff. This has been one of the most stimulating parts of my residency, a rewarding yet a difficult one.

Finally, I spent six months of my residency as a fellow at Barrow Neurological Institute in Phoenix (AZ) with Profs. R. Spetzler and V. Sonntag. This was a great experience since it offered me the opportunity to see another neurosurgical environment and to become involved in one area of their research.

I participated actively in the meetings of the Spanish Society of Neurosurgery by presenting papers. I also had the opportunity to attend some international meetings and a complete cycle of European courses. In spite of my overall satisfaction with my residency, there were some drawbacks: First, my training has been a clinical one. Even my research has been clinically oriented since there was too much work to find time for basic research. Second, grand rounds, journal club, and other academic sessions often interfered with the busy daily work, for instance the activity in the emergency department. Also, the impatience of the hospital authorities regarding the waiting lists often were a major cause of absence.

After this introduction, I would like to discuss three points, that in my opinion play an important role in the process of learning neurosurgery:

- The sources of neurosurgical information
- Learning to learn critically
- Travelling of the (young) neurosurgeon

Sources of Neurosurgical Information

During the residency it is extremely important to acquire a good theoretical basis and to incorporate new ideas and developments. This is as important as learning to move your hands in the surgical field. Sources of information are multiple, and except for a few selected exceptions, they are not written by residents or people in training. There is an increasing amount of neurosurgical information: textbooks, monographs, journals, videotapes, Internet, and so on. There are several fundamental textbooks of neurosurgery with regular new editions and updates. I have been ale to identify more than twenty journals directly related to neurosurgery, and Internet offers more than one hundred and thirty sources of interest for neurosurgeons [2].

For the individual resident several questions arise: Which sources of information should be available any time and everywhere? Which ones should be mandatory for the neurosurgiccal trainee? How to select reading, by whom? Can we attach reading and specific information to the training progress?

I tried to teach myself to select my reading but still I have no clear guidelines to offer. Often I succeeded in my selection, but many other times I read things which were outside my interest or my understanding, at least at the particular moment. Not infrequently a paper presented facts which completely opposed others, just recently read. It is diffuclt to decide which one is correct, particularly if a third publication some weeks later demonstrates that neither one was correct.

This fact stimulated Spanish residents to create their own journal, called NEUROCIRUGIA XXI, with residents being the main authors (Figs. 1, 2). Three types of papers are preferred: a) review of a given subject, b) bibliographical updates and c) anatomy cards. Senior neurosurgeons from Spain and from abroad are invited for specific articles and cooperation. The Editorial Committee is composed

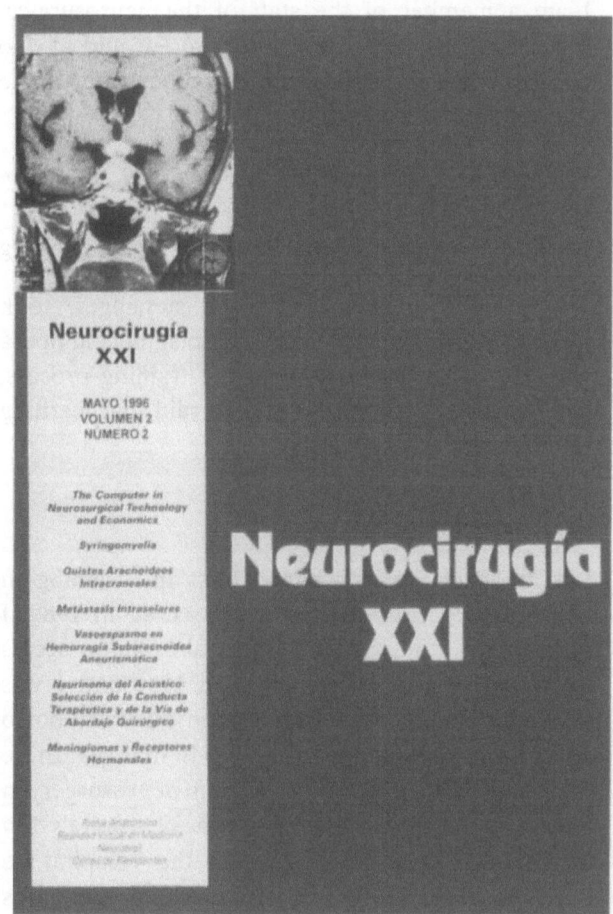

Fig. 1. Front page of "Neurocirugia XXI"

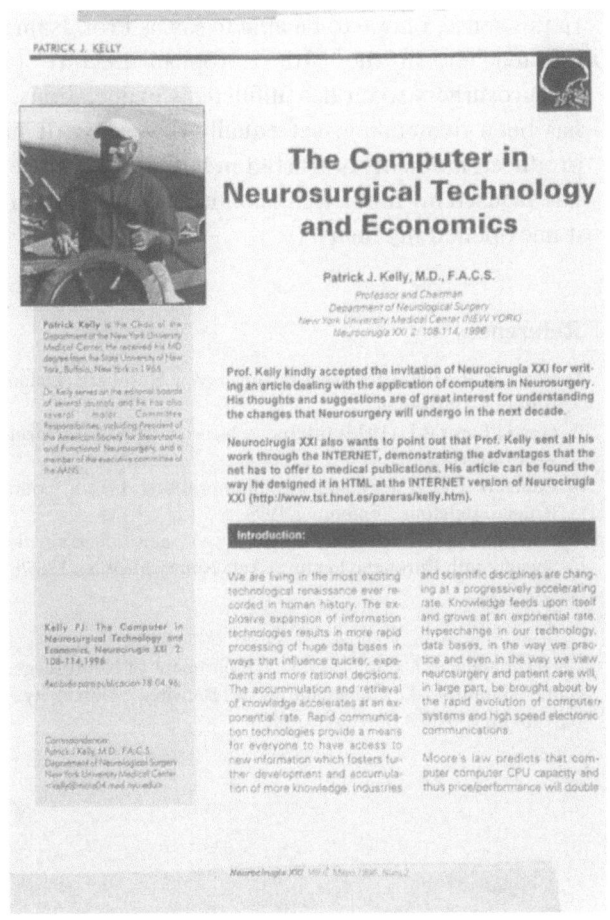

Fig. 2. Example of an invited article

of senior residents and junior neurosurgeons. The journal is sent free to any neurosurgical resident in Spain, and we are extending this offer to Latin America.

A careful selection of the sources of information is imperative, particularly during the first years of training. Therefore, trainees should be taught better to progressively choose their information and to develop solid criticism. Learning to choose is my second point of discussion.

Learning to Learn Critically

If learning to read critically is the main conclusion of my first point, this is just a part of the learning process: learning to learn critically is the basis for true learning. The capability to develop a critical approach and judgement is an important part of neurosurgical training.

Residents often spend their whole period of training in the same city, the same department, and under the same supervision. This means that they are exposed in a very specific way to practise neurosurgery; for example, one single way to perform a discectomy or to drain a chronic subdural haematoma. When doing things for a long period always in the same way, one may become seduced to believe that this is the only way to do it or even the only valid way. I consider this the "Single model of learning".

The use of therapeutic protocols is of great value in organizing clinical work as well as for evaluating final results. But they can refrain us from exploring other theraputic modalities. One must be aware that therapeutic protocols may play an unexpected role, namely to make us believe in one single way to do things.

Therefore, learning to become critical is one of the most difficult tasks for trainees, but is extremely important to reach a wide vision of neurosurgery. One must not be shy and the critical judgement should include all daily activities, even in the OR.

How does one learn to learn critically?
It is not a simple task but there are many ways to develop it: make comparisons, analyse results, including your own, travelling, attend meetings and conferences; remain flexible. I would like to remind of a sentence of Dr. Camaert [3], when he was asked about flexible or rigid endoscopy in neosurgery. He answered: "The endoscope should be rigid and the surgeon should be flexible."

There was one particular experience in my neurosurgical life that played a major role developing the necessary criticism: travelling.

The Travelling of the (Young) Neurosurgeon

I would like to focus briefly on the importance of travelling of the young neurosurgeon. Any resident should have the opportunity to spend some time outside his own department. It should be outside our country in order to see a completely different neurosurgical (and cultural) environment. It should be of adequate duration and probably be organized at a later stage of the training. Surgical inactivity during the travelling period is a major concern since toward the end of the training the resident should have maximum surgical activity, which can only be provided at the training hospital. Therefore, some good solutions must be found for the travelling as well as a stay abroad.

According to my experience I could identify many advantages, as for instance:

different ways to do things, use of different/new resources or techniques, knowledge of different departmental organizations, local differences in medical-legal aspects, local differences in ethics, new personal and professional relations.

On the other side, there are also some disadvantages: family and personal problems, financial problems, surgical inactivity at the end of the training period, being far from your country sometimes means to be far from job opportunities.

Conclusions and Suggestions

1. Residency is a period of learning that should inlcude learning habits of work as well as habits of thinking.
2. Developing critical judgement is one of the most important abilities that can be taught, encouraged and practised during the training period.

In this sense, I hope to be able to say as Prof. Isamat, my teacher, in the 17th European Lecture [4]: "Neurosurgery so far has fulfilled my expectations. It has been demanding, yet equally rewarding. It has produced moments of frustation but not of defeat. It has aroused my mind, it has conducted my hands and it has opened my heart."

References

1. Wagner R (1982) Die Meistersinger von Nürnberg. Daimon Editions, Barcelona
2. Garcia Pareras L (1996) Internet y Neurocirugià. Neurocirugià XXI (vol II):58–77
3. Camaert J (1993) Personal communications. FANS Course, Brugge, Belgium, September 1993
4. Isamat F (1996) Neurosurgery: an act of contrition. Seventeenth European Lecture. Acta Neurochir Wien 138:781–787

Correspondence: J. Cabiol, M. D., Department of Neurosurgery, Ciutat Sanitaria I, Universitaria de Bellvitge, University of Barcelona, E-08022 Barcelona, Spain

Acta Neurochir (1997) [Suppl] 69:79–82

"Control and Structure of a Training Program." The View of a Non-academic Hospital

J. Haase

Department of Neurosurgery, Aalborg Hospital, Aalborg, Denmark

Keywords: Neurosurgical training, non-academic hospital.

In order to discuss the view of a non-academic hospital, this term needs to be defined. A non-academic hospital is not a non-academic institution. The non-academic departments have all their staff being academics but lack – as compared to the university clinics – direct access to basic sciences institutes and to some extent medical students.

Do we actually witness differences between university clinics and non-academic hospitals in Europe today? It depends on who is looking and how the infrastructure of the hospitals has been developed. The university clinic is traditionally and historically based on basic science institutes and has the historic tradition of being the teaching hospital. In Denmark a non-academic hospital involved in neurosurgical training is considered to be at the same level as the university clinics. The presence of medical students creates a milieu with "academic" flavour composed of a variety of students and MD's on very different levels of education. Many non-academic hospitals are younger historically and medical students are often missing. Many of those hospitals in Europe are of private origin and proficiency is most important for their administration as it means survival or not. Therefore those hospitals have a tendency to appoint more senior MD's with a lesser degree of interest in science. Simultaneously the more humanity interested or dexterity oriented colleagues may be tempted to be functioning in such institutions as they see better chances here of performing without supervision by "scientists".

The university clinic is to a great extent involved in basic and clinical sciences with students working on theses or PhD programs in their departments contrary to what is found in the non-academic hospital. The medical students start their journey at university and may not see the non-academic institution until late in their studies or training. Therefore their images of what "medicine" or "neurosurgery" are may be distorted.

In order to become a neurosurgical specialist, a young Danish doctor starts with 18 months of basic training in medicine, surgery and psychiatry. Such positions are available in the majority of hospitals all over the country. However, the newly educated MD's are tempted to stay close to their initial institution and have their education in the university clinics.

Concerning neurosurgery we have five Danish institutions involved. Three university clinics in Copenhagen, Aarhus and Odense and two so-called non-academic institutions in Aalborg and Copenhagen County.

The Danish health authorities in their guidelines have recently made clear that they see no functional or educational differences between our five neurosurgical departments.

Education of a neurosurgeon is based on two facets – the personality training or development of medical competence behaviour and on the training of dexterity. Medical competence includes clinical judgment, medical knowledge, clinical skills, humanistic attributes, communication skills and continuing education. In order to become a neurosurgical specialist, the trainee must first accept a so-called *introductory position*, e.g. a position for one year in which the trainee is introduced to the speciality and can decide whether he/she wants to continue or not. Basically their tutor should also be involved in whether the trainee should or may continue but no official testing is required. The tutor's influence on deciding the credentials of the trainee is very limited – almost nil. If the introduction turns out favourably (as decided upon by the trainee) he/she can apply for *a two-year residency in neurosurgery*. In Denmark, three positions are available annually in our three university hospitals. Included in those positions is one year of neurosurgical and one year of neurology residency plus a 220 hour theoretical course on basic sciences and clinically related problems. A microsurgical three day course is also mandatory now. Following completion of his residency, the trainee will automatically-as part of the program-become *chief resident/senior registrar* for two years in one hospital and one year in another hospital. Following this, he/she will be certified as specialist in neurosurgery. There is no kind of examination or testing of knowledge or dexterity.

During the training the trainee has a personal tutor appointed responsible for the daily function. One of the heads of department is made responsible for the training program. Introductory, midway and evaluation talks are scheduled by the tutor and reported to the health authorities. Lately evaluation by an inspector of both the trainees and departments has been introduced, but is not in function. Yet, the tutor or the person responsible for education has no influence on the departmental daily function of their trainees. The workload is solely based on the will of the administration and the administrative head of the department.

The fact is therefore, that this program is not truly functioning today. The waiting time before the two-year residency is now around 5 years, and 7 months between introduction and residency. Before specialization results in a permanent position as "Oberarzt" or "Head", another 1–4 years of chief residency may be needed, depending on where in the country we are living.

Before 1981, a medical doctor in Denmark would work around 60–70 hours a week. Now the legal working time per week is 37.5 hours including on-call hours. A fixed schedule of rotation has been developed to secure these working hours. An example is

shown demonstrating that only during one week out of six, the resident will be involved in continuous clinical care of patient with potential possibilities of learning to operate. Until now some of the departments have used extra hours with overtime payment to create facilities necessary for education, but this has been stopped at present. In our department, since September it has been decided by our local authorities (hospital administration and county politicians) that all regulations must be followed due to lack of financial resources to pay overtime for the MD's. This means de facto that we have a resident attending during day time for nine days over a six week period in which elective surgical procedures can be performed in order to develop operative skills (dexterity). There will be 2 days for out-patient clinics and 2 days for work outside our department. The rest is free leisure time or on-call time. Therefore the local financial situation has great influence on education, something never even suggested in our national educational planning.

"Example is not the best method of teaching – it is the only method", stated Albert Schweitzer, but this has a hard time today in our managed care hospital environment with lack of confrontation time between trainee and teacher.

The greatest issue for medicine today in our high tech- and financially orientated societies is not that of proficiency but of humanity. Today due to high tech development, we can see patients leave the hospitals faster, in good health, cured of diseases that could not be treated earlier on. But our organisation and regulations, leaving the trainees as hour-to-hour slaves, with regulated working hours, long leisure time and computers to solve the patients' journey through the hospital, has left out the humanitarian aspects of medicine.

The values of active participation in our departments are greatly determined by us, the "Leaders". But it is the trainees that should be involved to a greater extent. In a Danish survey we could show that among the young residents a major part of their time was spent doing nothing or performing nonmedical work. This was also true to a lesser degree for the older, but both groups found that only a very limited part of their working time was of educational value. 34% of the daytime and only 4% of the on-call time for the chief residents was of educational value.

Teaching and learning is of course determined both by the teachers and the learners. Do we still accept that all teaching is based on teachers' decisions? – or should the learners be involved too? What is actually a teacher and what is an adult learner? What is a provider and a learner centred system?

A provider centred system has a syllabus, learning methods, pace of learning, time to learn and evaluation all selected by teachers, whereas economics is selected by politicians.

Learner centred programs are directed by the behaviour of adult learners. The adult learner is in control of his or her learning. He learns continuously, motivated by practice experience, and measures are taken by the learner himself, by impact on practice. Networks with peers are developed and he is motivated by peer comparison.

A contributor to performance is mental readiness, e.g. planned preparation activities, complete concentration and the ability to anticipate the next step. Distraction prevents a surgeon from staying alert, focused, relaxed and meticulous. Distraction control needs to be learned.

Surgery lends itself well to imagery for creating and rehearsing visual and tactile experiences such as transforming 2-D images from textbooks and X-rays into 3-D images of reality, rotating surgical procedures to suit various angles of entry, sensitizing oneself to the feeling of the tissue, to recognize when one has reached the right area, rehearsing procedural steps to facilitate more fluent and accurate movements, and to anticipate potential hazards and corresponding courses of action. Sincere bed side manners in doctor-patient relationship is developed as elite and experienced surgeons have listed consultation with the patients as a significant preparation activity.

Residents in neurosurgery may thus benefit from a more systematic training in mental skills just as the best athletes are doing.

With these reflexions we may begin to answer the question raised: "What is the view and the role of the non-academic hospital?" As already stated, according to the Danish health authorities no differences exist between the two hospital types. In Denmark, it is possible to have credentials as neurosurgeon without any training in a non-academic hospital or with only 25% of training spent in a university clinic. Egality does not prevail with this and is to me a severe mistake.

The university clinic due to its close collaboration with basic science institutes will develop programs for scientific work, PhD's and theses. Teaching in scientific methods is a natural part of the university training and the milieu creates a special scientific atmosphere. The intellectual process of learning to make decisions is difficult unless the role of apprenticing is accepted. We do still need this and the old British neurology model of reasoning beautifully demonstrates what can be achieved and what has been lost today to CT scans in the fight for efficiency. One hour of reasoning may be more valuable educationally than three wrong decisions made in a rush based on a superficial look upon some CT- or MRI scan. The university clinics should therefore have ample time to let this part of the training be a key factor.

In the non-academic hospital practical skills are more in focus. The two main reasons for surgical failures are either inferior decisions or most commonly errors in techniques during operations. This illustrates the possibilities of supplementary value of the two systems. Training in dexterity should be – and is to some extent – our basis in education. Dexterity is a simple eye-hand-brain reflex system, specific for human beings. Development of dexterity should be taught specifically in the non-academic institutions because practical skills are more easily developed there. A larger flow of basic patients and lesser number of specialists make the hands-on possibilities greater for the trainee. One point to remember is that teaching – unintentionally – is often neglected for the residents with least dexterity because it is more difficult and takes more time. Time for teachers is "money" wasted for administration. Fixed curriculum for hands-on training and supervision in training should therefore be mandatory. This training in our institution involves courses in microsurgery and foreign courses in St. Louis, USA, on skull-base surgery and Germany on endoscopy as part of our program for all senior registrars.

In the concept of a non-academic department, we must also teach our residents to be good learners, placing questions and be motivated to change form and format. Information without motivation can be obtained from computers but better professional care can only be added by motivation.

What for the Future?

A hospital with full training permission can be on different levels. The training of a neurosurgeon should never be carried out in a single institution. Differences among A- and B- institutions or university- and non-academic hospitals are therefore natural and a strength of a training system.

What about selection? The clinical practice needed is individually evaluated and selection of potential candidates must be considered more important than hitherto. Testing of personality and dexterity potentials before training and after completion of training should be a "must" today. Who would fly with a pilot that is not tested safe? Moral reasoning is a reliable predictor of clinical performance, whereas medical knowledge, grades and scores are poor predictors. In several papers the development of a superior surgeon is based on matching the correct personality and environment necessary to create an atmosphere which will germinate a concept of perpetual growth in knowledge and character. It has also been shown that a high level of moral reasoning virtually excludes a poor performance and that the highest level of clinical performance rarely is linked with a low level of moral. This selection and training could be a natural part of the job for the non-academic hospital and should be started during the introductory part of the training. The trainee should therefore have introduction in a non-academic institution only.

The non-academic hospitals should also produce dexterity training programs involving hands-on courses and computer based technical training. This combined with a sound basic apprentice type of teaching and teaching in personality development, will make the trainee fit for the more scientific and decision-making educational development being the key areas in the university departments.

A dedicated staff of teachers and program chairmen must be involved and this to me should not be the administrative heads of departments nor the professors, who should devote their time to scientific work of high standards. But we need written confirmation that training and time for education, both for teachers and learners, are part of daily life. If not, every time we cut down on function due to lack of financial resources, science and education will be hit.

Superspecialization has to be mentioned. Therefore the different institutions may be involved in European programs in order to provide necessary quality in training. This holds true especially for paediatric neurosurgery and stereotaxy.

What we also lack is a general EU level of training. Despite the UEMS suggestions, they have not been officially agreed upon in our countries. The necessity of education as part of MD function is not included satisfactorily in our daily life. A recommendation based on international suggestions would heartily be welcome by me. The American standards of teaching cannot be copied in Europe due to our diverse educational systems and historical traditions.

The role of the non-academic hospital in Europe will be specialization in dexterity training and close collaboration and linking of programs with a university clinic.

Correspondence: J. Haase, M.D., Department of Neurosurgery, Aalborg Hospital, DK-9100 Aalborg, Denmark

Acta Neurochir (1997) [Suppl] 69:83–88
© Springer-Verlag 1997

Assessment of Training Progress and Examinations*

J. T. Hoff[1] and **H. M. Eisenberg**[2]

[1] Section of Neurosurgery, University of Michigan Medical Center, Ann Arbor, MI and [2] Department of Neurosurgery, University of Baltimore, Baltimore, MD, U.S.A.

Summary

Board certification and accreditation of training programs began as measures of quality in the United States. Both functions were done initially by the American Board of Neurological Surgery (ABNS). In 1954, certification of trainees and accreditation of programs became separate functions in order to eliminate potential conflicts of interest.

Currently, the ABNS certifies trainees who have completed neurological surgery training in an accredited program whose curriculum includes operative and nonoperative experience, have the endorsement of the training program director, and have passed the written in-training examinations and a final oral examination. Accreditation of training programs is a separate function administered by the Residency Review Committee (RRC) of the Accreditation Council for Graduate Medical Education. Individual programs are reviewed on a periodic basis for quality of the curriculum, facilities, faculty, and patient volume. The ABNS and the RRC are separate groups, both comprised of neurosurgeons with a strong commitment to the educational process.

Keywords: Certification, accreditation.

Background

Neurosurgery became a subspecialty of surgery in the first decades of this century because of increasing interest in the nervous system and rapidly expanding knowledge about it. Harvey Cushing, an early pioneer of neurosurgery, recognized that "substantial improvement in neurosurgery would never be achieved until competent men restricted their work to that field alone" [3].

In the beginning, neurosurgical training was preceded by complete training in general surgery [7]. As time passed, training time shortened in general surgery and lengthened in neurosurgery. Training programs in neurosurgery began to appear. In 1920, Cushing and his colleague Ernest Sachs formed the first professional organization in our specialty, the Society of Neurological Surgeons [10]. The Society's purpose was to foster a healthy exchange of ideas in patient care, research, and teaching within the framework of good fellowship. There were twenty charter members in this group with an average age of 41 years. Only nine members had neurosurgery training that exceeded six months. Ten members, including Cushing, had no formal training but were exposed to neurosurgery during World War I or in clinics in the United States and abroad before the War. Two of the charter members of the Society were self-taught [11].

The American Board of Neurological Surgery (ABNS) was established in 1940 to develop standards of quality for the specialty in the United States. The ABNS was comprised of elected members from various societies that had formed within the specialty, including the Society of Neurological Surgery, with a mission to accredit training programs and to certify trainees from them. Fifty neurosurgeons were certified without examination initially. The Board continued to accredit programs and certify candidates through an oral examination process until the mid 1950s [6].

The accreditation of training programs and certification of their trainees by the same group (the ABNS) was perceived to be a conflict of interest within the specialty movement in the United States. In 1954, both the ABNS and the Council of Medical Education of the American Medical Association

---

* Drs. Hoff and Eisenberg have both served as Secretary and Chairman of the American Board of Neurological Surgery

(AMA) agreed that accreditation of programs should be separated from certification of trainees. A Residency Review Committee (RRC) for accreditation of neurosurgical programs was thus created under the joint sponsorship of the ABNS, the AMA, and the American College of Surgeons (ACS). The ABNS thereafter remained a separate and independent body, charged with examining and certifying fully trained neurosurgeons [8].

The Accreditation Council on Graduate Medical Education (ACGME) was formed in 1981. It was an agency of five parents (AMA, American Board of Medical Specialties, American Hospital Association, Council of Medical Specialty Societies, and Association of American Medical Colleges) that supervised the Residency Review Committees of all medical specialties. The ACGME was charged to standardize residency training in the various medical disciplines and to develop requirements for training.

The Residency Review Committee (RRC) for Neurosurgery was given the power through the ACGME to accredit programs based on periodic reviews of the curriculum developed by each, the availability of resources for training, the quality of the faculty in the program, and other specific requirements. Certification of trainees for programs accredited by the RRC was left to the ABNS where it had originated. The process for achieving high standards in the specialty that began in 1940 had thus separated quality control of the training program itself from the assessment of individual trainees within that program. The Director of the program assumed responsibility for the curriculum and all its resources. General and specific requirements were established nationally to provide consistency among the various programs. Requirements were periodically reviewed and revised by the Residency Review Committee, focusing on training essentials which included fundamental clinical skills, research opportunity, clinical neurology experience, basic science exposure, the length of training in each segment of training, the quality and quantity of the surgical experience and of the supervising faculty, and provision for progressive responsibility within the training process. The general aim of each Program was to provide an educational opportunity that would successfully train a safe and competent neurosurgeon within a reasonable period of time. The certification process evolved from an all-inclusive oral examination (1941–1970) to staged assessments consisting of passage of a written examination during training, successful completion of an accredited curriculum, two years of practice in the specialty, and finally an oral examination [6,9].

Current Assessment Process

Neurosurgery in North America continues to attract the best medical students. They are consistently well-rounded men and women who have excelled academically and stand at the top of their cells. Currently, three applicants in the United States compete for about every one position in the first postgraduate year. There are about 140 positions available annually [5].

Postgraduate Year I (Internship) Evaluations

Experience in fundamental clinical skills in the various surgical disciplines proceeds on a monthly rotation basis during the first year after medical school. Progress of the trainee is judged in writing by faculty and senior trainees on each service. Part III of the National Board of Medical Examiners (NBME) examination is taken near completion of the year. The trainee is required to pass before becoming licensed by individual states. Parts I and II of the NBME examination are taken during medical school; graduation requires passage of both Parts. Scores from each of the three Parts are provided to the trainee and to neurosurgery programs who have received applications for subspecialty training from each candidate.

Neurosurgery Resident Evaluations

Evaluations proceed on a semi-annual basis once the trainee has entered the formal neurosurgery curriculum. The evaluation includes a discussion between the Program Director and the trainee based on individual written assessments by the neurosurgery faculty members. Assessments by each faculty member are summarized anonymously. Progress of the trainee from year to year depends upon satisfactory completion of each year. Assessments are verified by both the Program Director and the trainee and are kept for the duration of the training period. Residents are appointed annually in the United States [2].

Resident Evaluation of Program

Residents are required to evaluate the curriculum of the program, and its faculty members annually for their teaching, clinical, and research skills. Resident evaluations of the program are given to the Program Director, who then may or may not provide anonymous evaluations to individual faculty members. The evaluation process of both trainees and faculty members thus enables them to critique each other and the program as a whole on a regular basis [2].

The Written Examination during Training

The National Board of Medical Examiners (NBME) provides a seven-hour written Primary Examination for residents in each program. Successful completion of the examination is required in order to complete the training program. Residents must take the examination at least once for credit during training, and they may take it yearly for practice and individual assessment of their progress through the training period [1].

The American Board of Neurological Surgery provides a pool of questions to the NBME in various categories from which each examination is constructed. The Primary Examination Committee consists of nine members of the Board. The examination is designed to test cognitive knowledge about neurosurgery. Examination questions fall into categories that include clinical neurosurgery, imaging, fundamental clinical skills and critical care, neuroradiology, neuropathology, neuroanatomy, and neurobiology. The examination contains 550 questions in various formats, often based on clinical scenarios. Each examination consists of new questions (67%) and old questions (33%) selected from a large pool of questions developed by the Committee. Old questions allow standardization of the exam so that each year performance can be compared to all other exams given in the past. The relevancy and effectiveness of each question as a testing tool is assessed after each examination by the NBME and provided to the Committee for its use as it develops the examination for the next year.

The pool of questions for the written examination is expanded annually by submission of questions by members of the American Board of Neurological Surgery and by other neurosurgical educators, including former Board members and training program directors who are not members of the Board. Individual questions are rejected by the Committee or edited in consultation with testing professionals from the NBME. The pass/fail score for the examination is determined using statistical comparisons. The validity of the entire examination, as well as each of the subsets, is also tested. The examination is proofread and edited by the members of the Committee after printing. Questions from each subtest are intermixed. After the examination, members of the Committee review the questions and responses, particularly questions with questionable statistics (for example, when quintiles scoring highest score lowest on a particular question). Some questions are withdrawn after discussion by the Committee, before final scoring is done.

The written examination is given annually in March. It is proctored by the Program Director. Security for the examination is stringent. Program Directors are forbidden to discuss questions with trainees in order to protect the purity of the pooled examination questions.

The NBME provides results of the examination to the Program Director, including performance of the trainees in individual test categories. This information allows the Program Director to adjust the curriculum on a regular basis whenever necessary. In addition, residents who take the examination are provided information about questions that were missed and categories of knowledge that should be improved. References are provided for each category so that the individual trainee can focus his or her study appropriately.

The pass rate for the examination is determined by the ABNS with the advice of the NBME. Sixty-four percent of questions correctly answered is the current minimum number required to pass. That percentage is remarkably consistent each year, indicating that the process is valid from year to year. Residents who are graduates of medical schools in the United States and Canada and are within two years of completion of training have a higher pass rate than others who take the examination for self assessment or for credit in the certification process.

Tracking Residents by the ABNS

The ABNS maintains a roster of individuals who are "tracking" for Board certification in individual programs. The progress of each resident is documented to maintain control of the number of residents in individual programs. That number should be the same as the number who are authorized for that program by the RRC. Disciplinary action of a program that exceeds the number of authorized residents may be taken by the RRC at the time of its periodic review. The ABNS maintains a list of Fellows and nonresident trainees in individual programs. Residents who withdraw or who are terminated from programs are also identified as a measure of the program and its interactions with trainees.

Program Director Letter to ABNS

Each trainee must have a letter of endorsement from the Program Director to the ABNS upon successful completion of the curriculum. Without the Program Director's endorsement letter, the trainee cannot proceed to oral examination.

Log of Individual Case Numbers During Training

A log of all operative cases for each trainee, whether as primary surgeon or assistant during the training period, is required by the ABNS before authorization for oral examination. The RRC requires the same data at its periodic review of individual programs, usually at intervals of three-to-five years.

Practice Experience

Practice experience for two years is required prior to oral examination. During that time, twelve months of practice data is recorded for both operated and nonoperated cases managed by the neurosurgeon during the period. Practice data may be assembled commencing three months after completion of the training program. A minimum follow-up period of three months for each case is also required. In addition, letters of endorsement from at least two neurosurgeons in the region who are aware of the performance of the neurosurgeon tracking toward certification are required prior to oral examination.

Credentials Review

The Credentials Committee of the ABNS (seven members) reviews each application for oral examination, including practice data, the Program Director's endorsement letter, and the endorsement letters of practicing neurosurgeons in the community where the candidate resides. The candidate is scheduled for oral examination by the Board upon approval by the Credentials Committee. The process currently requires about three years after completion of formal training before oral examination.

Oral Examination

The oral examination is given twice a year. Sixty to seventy-five candidates are tested during each examining session. The examination consists of three one-hour periods. The first concerns intracranial surgery, the second spinal and peripheral nerve surgery, and the third a combination of both. Examiners meet after the second-hour examination to discuss areas that have not been tested adequately during the first and second hours of examination. The examiners are Board members (14), former Board members (typically 2–3), and practicing neurosurgeons (15). Often neurosurgeons who are potential Board members are invited to examine in order to assess their skills as an examiner and to provide them testing experience.

Typically, case scenarios are presented to the candidate by two examiners for discussion. Hypothetical cases typify those seen in an average neurosurgery practice. Some neurological problems are also included. The question content is standardized as best possible so that the broad spectrum of the neurosurgery discipline is assessed. All of the examiners are clinical neurosurgeons. Their single purpose is to assess clinical judgment as accurately as possible.

All examiners meet to discuss individual performances at the conclusion of the three-hour examination. A numerical grading system identifies those who easily passed from those who clearly failed. Marginal candidates are discussed individually to determine their final grade. About 85% of those who are examined pass. Candidates are notified of the result the day following examination by letter. The Program Director of the examinee's program is also provided the same information. The performance of candidates for certification is provided to the Residency Review Committee regularly so that Programs can be assessed for quality based upon their residents' performance during the oral examination.

The Meaning of Board Certification in the United States

Certification by the ABNS has become a measure of quality, certifying successful completion of a curriculum of study including medical school, residency training in an accredited program, and successful performance on written and oral examinations. In reality, Board certification marks the successful completion of a well-defined curriculum designed to train safe and competent clinical neurosurgeons. Whether Board certification assures the quality of the trainee from that moment onwards can be debated [4].

It is possible to practice clinical neurosurgery in the United States without Board certification. Thus, of the 4,000 neurosurgeons practicing in the United States, only 3,500 are certified by the ABNS. The remaining 500 are not prevented from practicing the specialty by federal law protecting free trade. Thus, Board certification in the United States is not required for reimbursement of medical care.

Board certification increases the prospects for hospital credentialing and practice opportunity in the community. Most hospitals strongly encourage Board certification, but none are allowed to require it based on the restraint of trade concept inherent in American society.

Unresolved Issues

Standardization of the Oral Examination

Subjective and objective assessments of trainees must be as consistent as possible. Standardization of examinations to minimize bias by examiners is one approach to the problems of consistencies. Because much of the final oral examination is based upon clinical judgment, subjectivity is inherent in the process. Cognitive information is measured more easily by written examinations and by data, such as case logs and practice data review. The ABNS believes that the oral examination is a test of judgment and clinical performance, including on-the-spot evaluation of problems, including complications and expected outcomes.

While members of the American Board of Neurological Surgery believe that the oral exam is the best available method for probing clinical judgment and knowledge regarding the management of cases, this exam in its present context cannot be considered a standardized test because individual examiners use personal case material to develop the test scenarios. Thus, test material varies from examiner to examiner and from examination to examination. Individual examiners differ in their evaluations of the candidate's performance. Because of potential bias, some medical and surgical Boards in the United States have eliminated the oral examination, while others use duplicate question sets to reduce content and examiner variations to an absolute minimum. Members of the ABNS continue to believe that flexibility during the examination provides a method of probing both the candidate's capabilities and thought processes. The ABNS (with the help of an independent consultant) is currently developing statistical methods to weight difficulty of questions and severity of examiners within a flexible format for the examination.

Accreditation of Subspecialization

Most members of the American Board of Neurological Surgery subspecialize in their practice, but few advocate subspecialty certification. The ABNS believes certification in specific subspecialties threatens our small discipline with fragmentation and exclusivity, neither of which is desirable today. Some subspecialty groups, particularly pediatric neurosurgery, continue to advocate subspecialty certification, nevertheless.

Recertification

Presently, there are twenty-four Boards in various branches of medicine in the United States. All are members of the American Board of Medical Specialties (ABMS), a national organization that has fostered the Board movement for many years and provides a forum for discussion of problems that arise among the various disciplines. The American Board of Neurological Surgery began in 1940 and has been a member of the ABMS ever since.

The ABMS has endorsed recertification for three decades. Most of its Boards require recertification on a regular basis, including the American Board of Surgery, the American Board of Pediatrics, and the American Board of Internal Medicine. Those Boards believe that recertification is necessary to maintain safety and competency in an ever-changing world. Time-limited certification is a part of recertification. Typically, certification is granted initially for 7–10 years after which examination for recertification is required. Documentation of continuing medical education annually, written and oral examinations, and review of practice data for specific time periods are some measures used for recertification. Individual Boards of the ABMS have different recertification processes. The American Board of Neurological Surgeons is one of the few remaining that does not have a recertification process in place at the present time. The current position of the ABNS is that there is no testing process that measures safety and competence adequately, both of which are implied by recertification. The ABNS has preferred not to implement recertification until an instrument is developed that can accurately measure safety and competency.

Conclusions

The assessment of training progress and examinations in the United States and Canada has gone through an evolutionary process over the past 56 years. The process remains highly objective with periodic milestones that must be passed in order to continue towards certification. The final step in the process is an oral examination that tests clinical judgment and skills as measured by practicing neurosurgeons selected specifically for that process. In addition, the quality of the training programs from which candidates come is measured as objectively as possible by a separate group (RRC) whose purpose

is to focus upon the quality of the program and its curriculum.

References

1. American Board of Neurological Surgery Booklet of Information (1994, revised) ABNS, Houston, pp 18
2. Graduate Medical Education Directory, 1995–1996 (1995) American Medical Association, Chicago, Illinois, pp 1123
3. Fulton JF (1946) Harvey Cushing. Charles C Thomas, Springfield, pp 754
4. Hoff JT (1990) Subspecialty certification. In: Wilkins RH, Rengachary S (eds) Neurosurgery. Williams & Wilkins, Baltimore, pp 414–416
5. Hoff JT (1995) Neurosurgical education. In: Awad I (ed) Philosophy of neurological surgery, chapter 12. AANS Press, Park Ridge, pp 137–144
6. Kline DG (1990) Fifty years of service to American neurological surgery: The American Board of Neurological Surgery. Privately published, Houston, pp 102
7. Light RU (1992) Cushing's handwriting and remembering Harvey Cushing: the closing years. Surg Neurol 37:147–157
8. Mahaley JS Jr, Kline DG (1990) The American Board of Neurological Surgery: an historical perspective. In: Kline DG (ed) Fifty years of service to American neurological surgery: The American Board of Neurological Surgery. Privately published, Houston, pp 6–8
9. Pevehouse BC (1984) Residency training in neurological surgery, 1934–1984: evolution over 50 years of trial and tribulation. The 1984 AANS Presidential Address. J Neurosurg 61:999–1004
10. Sachs E (1958) Fifty years of neurosurgery: a personal story. Vantage Press, New York, p 186
11. Turnbull F (1984) As it was in the beginning. In: Alexander E (ed) History of the Society of Neurological Surgeons. 75th Meeting Anniversary. Hunter Publishing, Winston-Salem, pp 4–6

Correspondence: J. T. Hoff, M.D., Section of Neurosurgery, University of Michigan Medical Center, Ann Arbor, MI 48109-0338, U.S.A.

Acta Neurochir (1997) [Suppl] 69:89–92

Experience with the EANS Examinations

R. Braakman

Berkel-Enschot, The Netherlands

Keywords: European examination, experience, perspective.

Historical Development

The extensive experience with the USA Board Examinations, as presented, in the previous report, spans a period of 55 years; ours only 5 years.

After the second World War, quite understandably, it was not a simple task to accommodate people separated from each other by language, past history, religion and war, in one European Neurosurgical Society. Thanks to the pioneers, about whom you have already heard, the EANS was finally founded in 1971. Progressively and smoothly, English was subsequently accepted as a convenient language for scientific communication [1].

In January 1981, at a meeting organised by Jean Brihaye and attended by invited trainees, recommendations to improve quality of training were discussed. These recommendations were sent, in writing, to the national societies [2]. The expectations were that the recommendations might form a basis for future recognition of neurosurgical departments in the context of a European Board of Certification in Neurosurgery. The view of many members of the Administrative Council was that there should be a European Medical Association, which would require a European Certificate of Expertise from each medical specialist.

In 1982, during the course in Verona, it was proposed that trainees who had completed the entire five year cycle of courses should be invited to undergo an *oral assessment*. If successfully passed, the trainee obtained a diploma, the so-called European Certificate. The aim of this initiative was that one day, this examination, which was only a brief test, might develop into a real European examination at a higher level. Many of those who completed the 5 year course cycle took this examination.

In 1989, Mario Brock stimulated the creation of a committee in the EANS, with the aim to develop a European Examination comparable to those examinations provided by the American Board of Neurological Surgery.

A small committee of 7 people was formed, in which I acted as Chairman, and in 1991, it compiled a brochure containing recommendations and plans: "Towards a European Board of Neurological Surgery". These recommendations were accepted that same year by the Administrative Council.

The name of this committee was changed to *Examination Committee of the EANS*, because the designation, European Board of Neurosurgery had already been claimed by and reserved for the section of neurosurgery in the UEMS.

Its only task is to prepare and conduct the, to date voluntary, examinations. The Examination Committee has close connections with the Training Committee, which is primarily responsible for the training courses. Each committee has a different, though related task.

On several occasions I, and subsequently Jens Haase, have had the pleasure of being the guests of our American colleagues during the preparations for the primary examination and during the oral examination of the American Board. We were allowed to learn from their experience and could never have started our own project without their gracious help and support. We are particularly grateful to Mrs Sanderson, "Marie Louise".

We decided that we should not try to re-invent the wheel, but to follow more or less the program and format of the American examinations. Therefore, the actual *EANS Examination* consists of

a) a primary, written, multiple choice examination and
b) the final oral examination.

Actual Structure and Conduct of the EANS Examination

The first official *primary multiple choice examination* took place, after two try-outs, in Israel, just before the training course in September 1992. It was taken either as a first step towards the oral examination and certification, or for self-assessment. Subsequent primary examinations have been held once a year at the location of the annual European training course, just preceding it. Since 1994, for those not attending the course, it has also been held on the same day and at the same time in Brussels, thanks to the hospitality of Jacques Brotchi.

The primary examination is open to all residents in accredited neurosurgical programs in Europe and to all European certified neurosurgeons. Credit is not given to an individual who has worked in neurosurgery, without taking part in an official training program. He must obtain training as an enrolled trainee in an appropriate, nationally recognized program.

We advise that it is wise to wait until the fourth or fifth year of official training before taking the examination. Otherwise the examination is generally considered to be too difficult.

The primary examination consists of between 150 and 200 multiple choice questions. They are prepared by a primary examination committee, consisting of 7 program directors from different European countries. The analysis of the individual results is performed by the IMPP, the official German Institute for the design and analysis of examinations in Medicine and Pharmacy, whose office is in Mainz.

The examination includes questions on neurology, neuroanatomy, neurophysiology, neuropathology, neurology, neuroradiology, fundamental clinical skills and, of course, most questions concern neurosurgery. In the question 5 possible answers are provided of which one is correct, with possible answers always in alphabetical order. At this moment

Table 1. *Number of Applicants Primary EANS Examination 1992–1996*

Turkey	47	Hungary	13
Italy	41	Spain	11
Germany	25	UK	11
Netherlands	22	Switzerland	10
Scandinavia	17	Miscellaneous	65
Belgium	15		
Total	277		

Table 2. *Number of Applicants and Pass Rate Per Year*

Year	Number of applicants	Number who passed	Pass rate (in %)
1992	57	19	33
1993	61	32	52
1994	64	39	61
1995	52	32	62
1996	34	22	63

we have a stock of about 400 questions, which is far from the number required to gurantee completion of future examinations.

The original fee of 100 German Marks had to be increased to 200 German Marks in order to cover the costs of the analysis.

The distribution of the candidates according to country is shown in Table 1. The majority of the applicants from the UK are colleagues originating from the Middle and Far East. The French show only little interest in this exam. In striking contrast is the large number of Italian and Turkish colleagues. The percentages of those who pass (Table 2) per country are markedly in contrast to what many Western European colleagues express as their expectation.

The second and final step is the
Oral Examination:

The first oral examination was held in Brussels 2 years ago. This year we had the third oral examination, unfortunately with very few candidates. I shall discuss this point later. The Oral Examination is the second and final of the European Examinations. A pass at the Oral Examination is the only way of obtaining the European Certificate in Neurosurgery.

The requirements to take part in this examination are:

– evidence that the primary European examination in neurosurgery has been passed.

- license to practice neurosurgery in any European country. A copy of this license must be forwarded for inspection.
- at least two years of practice in neurosurgery as an officially licensed neurosurgeon in any European country.
- a log book of operations, independently performed during a consecutive period of 12 months after the license was granted.
- advance payment of the fee payable in German Marks as specified on the application form. This was 1,200 German Marks, but has, this year, been reduced to 800 German Marks.

The examination in the english language consists of three parts, each lasting one hour:
The first hour is dedicated to an oral examination by two examiners on operative neurosurgery of brain and skull. In the second hour operative neurosurgery of spine, cord and peripheral nerves is covered. In the third hour the topics to be discussed are those that could not be adequately covered in the first two hours.

The examination is a clinical problem solving and patient management test. It is not a theoretical examination, like the primary examination. Case histories are given, and appropriate X-rays, scans, MRI's, and other visual aids are shown to augment the presentation and development of cases.

Candidates explain verbally how they would proceed to evaluate or manage the cases and to plan and perform the proposed operations, if indicated. A sufficient number of models of skull, brain, spine and peripheral nerves is available. Four to six cases are discussed per hour.

Each of the three hours is conducted in an interview setting with two examiners, experienced neurosurgeons from a European country.

During these three hours, therefore, the candidate will meet six different European examiners, each of whom gives an independent score. The final, combined score is available the same day. A candidate who receives a pass grade for this examination will be granted the European Certificate of Neurosurgery.

It is our intention that the level of our examinations should be comparable to the level of the Examinations of the American Board of Neurological Surgery. Perhaps we have not yet achieved this expectation. This remark applies in particular to the primary examination. In the USA it now consists of

540 multiple choice questions and includes microscopic pathology specimens. We still wonder why there should be so many questions.

Those of us who have attended or participated in the oral examinations on both sides of the Atlantic, share the view that our examinations are at least comparable to the level of the American exams.

Misunderstandings about the European Certificate

Many former trainees who have passed the oral assessment at the end of the European training course and obtained a diploma, believe that the present European (EANS) Examination is the same as, and simply a continuation of, this post-course assessment. This is not correct. The EANS Examination, consisting of two parts, is far more difficult and of a far higher level than the previous brief test at the end of the course. It is much more difficult to pass.

The other misunderstanding is the belief that this European Certificate gives the right to practice neurosurgery in any European country, or in an EC country. This is a major misunderstanding. The European Certificate does not replace any national license. It is an award rather than a license. The Certificate reveals that the owner has a good level of theoretical and practical knowledge in the field of neurosurgery and should increase his/her chance of obtaining a good position.

Opposition to a European Certificate

The concept of a European Certificate has met with much opposition from members of various national societies. They are afraid that colleagues from another country, perhaps certified at a different level (correctly or incorrectly considered to be a lower level) would be able to start practice as a neurosurgeon anywhere in Europe because they have this Certificate.

Many European colleagues are afraid that their country will be inundated by neurosurgeons with this Certificate from elsewhere in Europe and are even more concerned about an influx from Asia and Africa.

This concern is unnecessary, at least for the moment.

The requirement for participation in the oral examination is that the candidate should hold a national license to practice neurosurgery. Once again, the European Certificate is not a license. It is an award.

No one who has been involved, either as candidate or examiner, has so far expressed negative feelings about the examinations. In particular the colleagues who examined during the time consuming and fatiguing oral examination were quite enthousiastic and willing to participate the following years again, although there was no financial compensation whatsoever for the days involved.

There are, however, also critical remarks.

James Palmer, for instance, the Editor of Neurosurgery 96, remarks: "If I do not need to pass an examination which will cost me a fair amount of money to take, why should I put myself through the humiliation if I fail?" [3]

In contrast, Mrs Cesarini from Sweden, who was one of the first to take and pass the examination, states in another chapter of this book: "Courses and congresses are excellent, but we need to prove ourselves that we can maintain a certain standard. Being examined by six different senior neurosurgeons from all over Europe guarantees a fair examination and an interesting discussion. The examination does not give us any legal rights, but by working on it and improving it, it will become a very effective tool to influence training, improve exchanges across Europe and make our profession strong and competent. Soon the legal aspects will change, and there will probably be a long queue of neurosurgeons waiting to be examined. No need to state that I fully agree with this view." [4]

Still my concerns are:

1. the number of candidates for the primary examination is sufficiently high, but is slowly decreasing. I do not know why.
2. the number of applicants for the oral examination remains disappointingly small, about 10 per year. Some potential candidates, who met the requirements, claimed that the fee, which is only a frac-

tion of the American fee, is far too high, in particular for Eastern and some Southern European countries. Therefore, we reduced the fee from 1,200 to 800 German Marks, and this year, by mistake, to 400 German Marks, but the number of applicants did not increase.

Another criticism is that the examination does not test manual dexterity. This is true, but the statement that that aspect "is the only aspect that really counts" is not true. The fact that dexterity cannot be tested does not imply that all other aspects should not be tested either.

In my view the goal of this examination was and is: to be a tool in attempts to improve the standard of neurosurgical training in those parts of Europe where this is necessary, and where there are no nationally organized examinations. This goal will never be achieved without strong support from the national Neurosurgical Boards, their training committees and the national representatives in the training committee. We have acquired expertise and experience; it would be a pity if this is lost.

However, the decision whether we should or should not continue and intensify the examinations has to be taken soon by our national representatives in the executive committee of the EANS.

References

1. Brihaye J (1984) History of the European Association of Neurosurgical Societies. Neurosurgery 15:262–264
2. Brihaye J, Brock M, Isamat F, Garfield J, Vigouroux R (1983) Assessment of neurosurgical departments and training in neurosurgery. Conclusions of a symposium in Brussels 1981. Acta Neurochir 68:171–174
3. Palmer J (1996) In: Palmer J (ed) Neurosurgery 96. Manual of neurosurgery. Churchill Livingstone, p 13
4. Cesarini KG (1996) The European Examination. The candidate's perspective. In: Palmer J (ed) Neurosurgery 96. Manual of Neurosurgery. Churchill Livingstone, p 14

Correspondence: Prof. Dr. R. Braakman, Udenhoutseweg 10, 5056 PE Berkel-Enschot, The Netherlands

Acta Neurochir (1997) [Suppl] 69:93–97
© Springer-Verlag 1997

Experience with the United Kingdom Examinations in Neurosurgery

J. D. Pickard*

Academic Neurosurgical Unit, University of Cambridge, Addenbrooke's Hospital, Cambridge, United Kingdom

Summary

The UK Intercollegiate Specialty Board examination in Surgical Neurology was established in 1991 based on the experience of the original Royal College of Surgeons of Edinburgh Assessment in Surgical Neurology, an exit examination that was originally opposed both by surgery in general and by the younger neurosurgical community. Criteria for eligibility encompass both UK, EC and non-EC overseas graduates. Candidates must have completed satisfactorily their 4th year of a 6 year training programme, have personal experience with the more straightforward benign tumours, aneurysms and posterior fossa explorations, and be able to safely manage a conventional neurosurgical practice. The examination consists of a multiple choice question paper, clinical examination and three Vivas. A curriculum is under construction. Examinations are held twice per annum, and rotate between the four colleges. There are strict guidelines for the examiners. The pass rate is about 70%. All aspects of the examination continue to evolve and are carefully audited.

Keywords: Neurosurgery, examination, training.

Historical Background

At the risk of causing offence, it is illuminating to consider the history of the introduction of a neurosurgical examination in the United Kingdom. The medical profession in general and surgery in particular remains obsessed with examinations, an enthusiasm not shared by other professions, nor reflected in their inferior standards.

"Perfect happiness for student and teacher will come with the abolition of examinations, which are stumbling-blocks and rocks of offence in the pathway of the true student".

Sir William Osler, 1899 [1]

Inspection and accreditation of neurosurgical training took many years to become established and accepted in the United Kingdom with the inevitable change from apprenticeship to a more structured approach to training. Whereas the younger generation was in favour of such inspection, the concept of a neurosurgical examination, muted by the Royal College of Surgeons of Edinburgh in the 1970's, was vigorously opposed by the Neurosurgical Senior Registrar Association, not least because the examination was to be imposed sans curriculum, sans training/teaching courses, sans educational objectives.

Senior Registrars during the early 1970's of whom I was one, considered that too much time had already been squandered on excessive training in general surgery in order to gain the obligatory FRCS. At the age of 28 years, one was free to return to Osler's true path and pursue Neurosurgery. Far from an attempt to rationalize, evaluate or excise the irrelevant and often capricious elements of the existing examination structure, here was an initiative by the soon – to – be – retired generation to shackle young minds with yet anothe hurdle. There was scepticism about the motives. Was it an attempt by the Royal College of Edinburgh to generate income? Was it the desire of the older generation to create a comfortable travelling dining club? Where was the evidence that training would be improved by such an examination? What deficiencies had been identified in the older generation to justify it? What would be the implications for time available for original research? Was it

---

* Current Chairman of the Intercollegiate Board in Surgical Neurology (U.K.). Opinions expressed in this article are those of the author alone and should not be taken to represent those of the Intercollegiate Board

simply an attempt to emulate the American Board, given the slow devaluation of the General Surgical FRCS, even though there was no intention to encourage free movement medical manpower across the Atlantic – quite the contrary.

Not surprisingly, the UK Senior Registrars successfully boycotted the examination for a few years. The standard to be expected was claimed verbally to be that of an experienced registrar moving straight from the ward and operating theatre to the oral/clinical examination. However it was not long before tales emerged of examiners asking obscure basic neuroscience questions of no clear relevance to clinical care.

This historical account is in part a caricature that may induce outrage in some quarters but does reflect the passions aroused at the time. The early pioneers of the examination – Professor Gillingham, Mr. Gordon and Mr. Miles Gibson – understood the shortcomings of the Edinburgh initiative but persevered against the conservative force of general surgery and the differing opinions of the four separate Royal Colleges of London, Dublin, Glasgow and Edinburgh. The first Specialty Assessment in Surgical Neurology of the Royal College of Surgeons of Edinburgh was held in 1977 and the first Intercollegiate Board examination in 1991. It represented a welcome bringing together of the four Royal Colleges with the Society of British Neurological Surgeons.

Intercollegiate Specialty Board in Surgical Neurology

The UK neurosurgical community is blessed by being able to use the umbrella provided by the comprehensive facilities of the Intercollegiate Board based in Edinburgh with access to the experience of all the other surgical specialities through regular meetings of the Joint Committee on Intercollegiate Examinations of the Senate of Surgery of Great Britain and Ireland. The Surgical Neurology Board is always composed of representatives of each of the four Royal Colleges of Surgeons (Dublin, Edinburgh, Glasgow and London), two Representatives from the Society of British Neurological Surgeons and the Chairman of the Specialty Advisory Committee (SAC) in Neurosurgery (who cannot be the Chairman of the Examination Board). The SAC is responsible for inspecting all training programmes and

monitoring of progress of all trainees, both home and overseas. There has been a fundamental restructuring of training in the United Kingdom – so called Calmanisation. All training programmes for Specialist Registry in Neurosurgery are now 6 years in length as detailed elsewhere in this volume by Mr. Hide and Mr. Shaw.

Eligibility

Much discussion continues over the flexibility of the criteria for eligibility for the examination. It is wasteful of the examiner's time and unfair to applicant's bank accounts to allow uncompetitive candidates to proceed. The examination currently costs £500 rising to £600 over the next year.

Curriculum

No detailed curriculum has ever been published although a draft was produced by the late Professor

Table 1. *Regulations Relating to the Specialty Examination in Surgical Neurology*

1. The candidate must hold a medical qualification recognised for registration by the General Medical Council or the Medical Council of Ireland and must have been qualified for at least seven years.

2. The candidate must hold a basic surgical training diploma of one of the Royal Surgical Colleges of Great Britain and Ireland (ERCS or MRCS/AFRCS (awarded from 1998) or an equivalent diploma formally recognised by the Colleges.

3. The candidate must have completed satisfactorily four years of higher training in the specialty acceptable to the relevant Board.
a) Candidates who are training with a view to award of the Certificate of Completion of Specialist Training (CCST) by the Specialist Training Authority or the Medical Council of Ireland must have enrolled with the relevant Specialist Advisory Committee (SAC) and completed these four years of training within a programme approved by the SAC. A satisfactory fourth-year assessment will be required.
b) All other candidates must have spent at least one of these four years in a training programme in Great Britain or Ireland approved by the relevant SAC, the mandatory year offering experience equating to fourth-year level within the specialist registrar grade. A satisfactory fourth-year assessment will be required. Candidates must have written confirmation from their trainers that the mandatory year of training will be at fourth-year level. Any other training done in Great Britain and Ireland must have been in posts approved by the relevant SAC. With regard to training undertaken outwith Great Britain or Ireland, it will be helpful to the Board in assessing its acceptability to have the candidate's record of operative experience over this period. The decision of the Board shall be final.

Table 2. Examination Scope and Format

Candidates are expected to be fully conversant with all aspects of neurological surgery.

Candidates will require a sound knowledge of clinical practice, investigation, diagnosis, management and the standard operative procedures in Surgical Neurology.

Candidates will require a detailed knowledge of the Basic Sciences as applied to Surgical Neurology.

The format of the Examination will be:

1. An MCQ in Basic Sciences applicable to Surgical Neurology.
2. A one-hour clinical examination conducted in a clinical setting.
3. Three half-hour orals in each of the following:
   a) Operative Surgery and Surgical Anatomy
   b) Investigation of the Neurosurgical patient including Neuroradiology
   c) The non-operative practice of Surgical Neurology which includes Intensive Care and the clinically applied Basic Sciences.

LOG BOOKS

Log Books must be brought by the candidate to the Oral Examinations.

The Norman Dott Medal

The above medal will be awarded annually by the Board to the candidate(s) who has the most outstanding performance in the examination during that year.

Douglas Miller after due consultation in 1990. There had been fears that questions asked about topics not included in the curriculum might lead to appeal and litigation. Such concerns have now been addressed and a general curriculum is under construction. The current guide to the scope and format of the examination includes the following (Table 2).

The MCQ is under review and may be replaced in party by a Spot examination that is more flexible and makes creation of a copy database more difficult.

Frequency of the Examination

Two 'diets' of the examination are held per annum and rotate between the four Royal Colleges. However, each College may delegate the location of the examination to a teaching hospital so that examinations have been held for example in Cambridge, Liverpool and Birmingham.

The Examiners

There is an annual advertisement for application to the Panel of Examiners. Candidates should have at least 7 years experience as a Consultant in active National Health Service practice in a unit accredited for training and have a satisfactory curriculum vitae. Most of the examiners are Neurosurgeons but the panel also includes Neuroradiologists and Neuro-intensive care specialists. Examiners serve for 5 years with possible re-election for 2 to 5 years after a gap year, depending on the actuarial statistics for the specialty. There is no formal training as an Examiner except for attendances as an Observer at one examination and subsequent pairing with a more experienced colleague. However there are strict guidance notes for examiners, for marking and for adjudication that are rehearsed at the start of every examination in the light of experience. No examiner may examine any current trainee nor any potential appointee to their unit. Examiners must declare any interest in any candidate. Great care is taken with the marking schedule to avoid inappropriate debate at the time of adjudication. Examiners are unaware of marks achieved in other parts of the examination by an individual candidate. A running log is kept of topics discussed to ensure that as wide a range of topics as possible is covered. Over the course of the examination, a candidate will be seen by 8 different examiners.

Standard and Pass-rate

To be successful a candidate must convince the examiners that they are able to manage safely a conventional neurosurgical practice. Examiners are asked to avoid detailed questions on their sub-specialty interest. At the end of 4 years training, candidates should have personal experience of the more straight forward supratentorial benign tumours, aneurysms and posterior fossa explorations and have the confidence of their trainers as reflected in a satisfactory end of 4th year assessment as confirmed by the SAC.

Since April 1991, the overall pass rate has been 70% (range 33–100%) with between 1–17 candidates/examination.

Some Problems

Distraction from Original Research

This examination seeks to establish safety. Is the candidate competent now and does he have the appropriate humility and personality to recognise this hurdle as simply an episode in the natural development of their lifelong education and training? Will they remain open to new knowledge yet critical in its application? Unfortunately there is ample evidence that this examination is deflecting young neurosurgeons from their original research with declining competition for prize competitions and failure to complete theses for higher degrees at an age when they are at their most productive [2]. The Board sets a high priority in ensuring that the format of the examination is focussed on clinical competence and a working knowledge of *relevant* neuroscience. The MCQ is under continuing review to make sure that it is unambiguous and seeks out clinically relevant knowledge.

Eligibility and Flexibility

With the introduction of a 6 year training programme, the criteria of eligibility have been crystallized both for EC and overseas candidates. Despite the apparent clarity of these eligibility criteria, problems may arise. It is essential that trainees, particularly from overseas, have written confirmation when they have entered the critical fourth year of training and when their end of 4th year training assessment will be. That assessment is conducted internally both by local neurosurgeons and representatives of the Post Graduate Dean. It is the responsibility of the SAC to confirm to the Intercollegiate Board that a satisfactory 4th year has been completed, together with confirmation of periods of Higher Surgical Training for which eligibility to sit the examination is claimed. Only then is the Intercollegiate Board able to accept an application to sit the examination. Pleas for flexibility often reflect failure by either trainee, trainer, or both to attend in advance to these simple requirements. It is too little understood that the examination is but one part of the packsge – training, education, assessment – to mark successful completion of standard neurosurgical training prior to subspecialisation. It is not in the candidates best interest to be allowed to sit for the examination before he is ready, not least because of the expense. A trainer may, out of misplaced loyalty, write an over optimistic assessment that simply leads to failure and loss of £500 plus.

Examiners

Candidates will be at least 30 years of age and rightly will be intolerant of any amateurism in the conduct of an examination that is crucial to their future careers. It is incumbent on the Examination Board to try and ensure that their examiners are neither hawks nor doves but sympathetic, experienced diviners of clinical competence in their future colleagues. Much discussion now centres on how to induct examiners and how to create a common code of conduct. Fortunately the introduction of such a mechanism is being pursued in advance of any problems occurring and not in reaction to any past lapses. Examiners need to be part of the creation of the MCQ and spot questions to be aware of the standard expected in the basic neurosciences and investigations. Examiners may even choose to sit the examination first! Within a decade, most examiners will themselves have passed the examination but will still need to be brought up to date with regard to both its content and philosophy.

Validation

Almost certainly the UK Intercollegiate Examination will undergo iterative validation in consulation with educationalists expert in clinical assessments over the next few years under the overall umbrella of the Joint Committee of the Royal Colleges. It is essential that an examination at such an advanced stage of training is perceived to be relevant, fair and professionally orchestrated, not least because of the legal consequences of sloppy procedures.

Conclusions

The UK examination is about defining competence, safety and the ability to incorporate new knowledge over a professional life time. In a sound training programme, trainers and trainees should learn together. Examinations should not be a capricious hurdle that will deflect the trainee from the much more important and imaginative path of original observation and innovation that has served Neurosurgery so well for so long. Certainly my personal impression, unsubstantiated by any official statistics, is that the level of excellence in the examination does not correlate with subsequent progress, academic innovation or medical legal complications! Let us hope that John Hunter's view of another ancient university never applies to this examination; "they wanted to make an old woman of me but these schemes I cracked like so many vermin". There is little sympathy in the United Kingdom for the view that examinations should form part of continuing medical education.

Acknowledgements

I am deeply indebted to Mr. M. Gibson for his insight into the establishment of the Intercollegiate Examination and to Mrs. E. Winton of the Intercollegiate Board for her unfailing advice and efficiency with running the examination. All inaccuracies and prejudices are the sole responsibility of the author.

References

1. Osler W (1905) Counsels and ideals from the writings of William Osler
2. Pickard JD (1993) Threats to academic neurosurgery. J Neurol Neurosurg Psychiatry 56:1143–1148

Correspondence: J. D. Pickard, Academic Neurosurgical Unit, University of Cambridge, Box 167, Level 4, Addenbrooke's Hospital, Cambridge CB2 2QQ, United Kingdom

Acta Neurochir (1997) [Suppl] 69:98–100

Periodic Evaluation of Training Progress and Teaching

M. Vapalahti

Department of Neurosurgery, University Hospital, Kuopio, Finland

Keywords: Neurosurgical training, Evaluation of teaching, Examinations Training program.

Introduction

The subject of this presentation is not outside evaluation of the training process, which certainly is one possibility for improving the quality of training, even if perhaps expensive and bureaucratic. The subject rather is the normal, continuous, honest and internal audit of the education process, a more practical and effective method. Actually "education" is the word I would like to use for the training process of a neurosurgeon.

Undoubtedly the selection criteria for residents in Neurosurgery are the starting point of the training progress evaluation: at which level do we begin, what is the motivation. Colleagues, trained mainly during the 60's were selected in many different and peculiar ways, as described in previous chapters. I have one story to add. I was picked up as a promising young trainee during the department's weekend trip to my boss's summer place in the Helsinki archipelago. All the juniors had to try waterskiing, with our professor at the helm. I did that quite well, on the first try, it was not that much different from cross country skiing, and I received the training position.

How was I educated? With a lot of clinical work and overwork. On call every second night; if not neurosurgery, then anesthesiology. No social life, always tired and on parties known to drop off to sleep immediately after the welcome drink. There were no good textbooks yet in the 60's; neurosurgical journals seemed to handle irrelevant problems; there was no money for congresses; and meetings were there only if you organized them yourself. But on the other hand you had an unlimited number of patients to investigate, to operate, to take care of. You got good advice from colleagues and a hand during the operation if needed – with some gentle hazing. There was increasing motivation to learn more, and good mentors. That was neurosurgical education; it could have been much better.

Requirements

L. Calliauw already presented the European model of the training program, a work of the UEMS [1]. The training program must be generally accepted, and minimum quality standards are set for teachers, operations, equipment and connections to other branches of medicine. More important in this context is the teaching program. There should be a clear, comprehensive program for each year that is, written but still flexible. The criteria for acceptance into the teaching program should be open and public, and in the follow-up the trainee's logbook is mandatory part of the follow-up. The minimum number of operations to be attended is 600 in 4 years, and personal operations should be performed on at least 135 patients.

The program must also include possibilities for independent active learning, and it must be financially sound. We should not forget that the young residents working during the more difficult hours of the day and night are bringing in a great amount of money to our teaching departments, at least one third of our department's 15 million DM budget. The rights of the trainees should be considered when planning the program. The requirements of young trainees in the response of the Finnish Medical Association to

Table 1. *What Trainees in Finland want from Their Program*

– a personal tutor
– independent learning
– assisted operations
– time out to read
– own research program

the new European Medical Specialist Directive are quite the same as what we are suggesting now (Table 1).

The training program should be research oriented, meaning, that it should also be connected with a university. This provides trainees with the possibility to learn together and from each other, and I think that competition should not be the main source of energy. Time after the training should also be a concern of the teachers, before accepting the residents, during the teaching and especially at the end of the training period.

Evaluation

Training programs should be inspected regularly, this happens already in the US and the UK, and there is a plan for the UEMS. The central register should have all the written programs, and a team of (three) teachers should visit the place each 5th year. Usually, the teaching center itself requests the evaluation and takes care of the costs. At least one (chairman) should be from another country, and before the visit an internal audit should be performed to answer standardized questions; this can be the starting point for the external audit. A visit should not last longer than a day, and the written report should be finished within 4 weeks.

Individual training progress can be much more difficult to assess. At the end of the training period, formal evaluation is of course mandatory in most countries. It can be at first local, but soon national for specialist degrees or European as standardized by the EANS. This EANS examination is multiple-choice type, like many national tests. The Finnish examination is an essay-type, based on textbooks, the preceding 4 years' neurosurgical journal knowledge, and relevant basic research.

During training, evaluation may be continuous, and will be performed more or less intentionally by the faculty and program leader. A periodic cognitive evaluation is also possible; a much better method would be self-evaluation. The problem with evalua-

tion is that we are dealing with highly educated, motivated young adults, with a mean age of 27–32 years, who are in different phases of their training and skills. The other problem is knowing what we should or can evaluate in young neurosurgeons: manual skills, clinical abilities or character. Theoretical knowledge is the only single area for which we have tests and different qualities to analyze.

Oral Evaluation

I have difficulty seeing much use for periodic annual examinations during training. Actually all teachers know, that they themselves can be the worst obstacles to learning. A larger team facilitates easier communication, and the personal, sometimes emotional problems of teaching can be partly avoided. Teaching at this level is always mostly communication, and the teacher needs feedback as well. The requirements of the program include that the program leader should be available most of the time in the teaching institute. An important possibility is oral evaluation, annually or twice a year. A preplanned, programmed timing is needed in an undisturbed place with a fixed (2–3 hours) time schedule.

The logbook, which the trainee has filled out during the evaluation period is extremely important. It may be kept by the trainee, but it should be easy to compare with the department data statistics. Problems in fulfilling the requirements of the planned program should be discussed first, then the other aspects of operative and clinical work: is there a need for more assistance, special cases, own operations? What are the plans for the next period? Problems in learning should be discussed, as well as department meetings and outside courses. The goals of the trainee, the timing of the education and research goals should also be part of this discussion. The need for reading, writing and self-assessment should be planned; this often means time out of clinical work.

More personal things can be included in this discussion, but only on the terms of the trainee.

Evaluation of Character

I am quite sure that it is not necessary to clone our residents into identical profiles during their neurosurgical education. But do we have to accept all the flowers? The most difficult thing to evaluate, and actually impossible to treat are problems of character, especially unethical behavior. This is not easy to define legally, but it is in fact a very clear weakness to deal with in such a vulnerable and confidential atmosphere as is found in a teaching hospital. If there is a suspicion of unethical attitude, one should listen carefully, but not ask the team, personnel, patients and other trainees. Real moral problems are incurable, and if you have to terminate a career, do it early. Before such a decision, senior members of the team should know the lines of argument. Discussion of the matter is of course the right of the trainee. Confidential discussion of the legal aspects with the hospital attorney is useful, but the decision is the program leader's alone, and is emotionally more difficult than an unnecessary complication in an easy craniotomy.

Conclusion

It could be useful to remember, that at this time of laws limiting extra working hours everywhere in Europe, it is not necessary for trainees in such a specialty like neurosurgery to become tired and burned out. Learning takes energy; this should be used economically. On the other hand, one-third of neurosurgery must be handled and learned acutely. The speciality needs women; equal rights and working flexibility are part of that decision. Bringing up children is a lifetime duty for men as well. There is not only life before death but even before board examination. Good training programs must provide reasonable free time for junior neurosurgeons, even a break for research.

The new generation of neurosurgeons must remember that their education is dependent (as it has always been) mostly on their own motivation and initiative. That's why they must learn to share their work better, to be a better team and to grow together.

References

1. Calliauw L (1997) The UEMS model of neurosurgical training. Acta Neurochir (Wien) [Suppl] 69:75–79

Correspondence: M. Vapalahti, M.D., Department of Neurosurgery, University Hospital, FIN-70210 Kuopio, Finland

Acta Neurochir (1997) [Suppl] 69:101–105
© Springer-Verlag 1997

What Consequences Should Result from Failure to Meet Internal Standards?

J. Schramm

Department of Neurosurgery, Bonn University Medical Center, Bonn, Federal Republic of Germany

Summary

This paper tries to approach a difficult problem, namely how to deal with a resident who has failed to meet the internal standards of a residency training program. First the problems of the definition of a standard and the associated problems of its reproducibility, documentation, teaching, update, and internal variability inside the same teaching program are dealt with. Consequently the question needs to be answered that constitutes a failure to meet the standard. The results of a survey of residents' attitudes are quoted as are some responses to a survey among the chiefs of teaching programs. Considering the attitudes of residents on how to handle breaches of standard the basic message was that residents want to be told that they do not function. Both parties want the collaboration of senior staff members on this topic. Whereas residents want to re-train, exercise and talk they do not want sanctions. Chiefs, however, want much less re-training, exercising and talking but earlier sanction. The difficult point of dealing with a true failure is discussed in the light of the German legal situation and the actual possibilities of how to handle the case. Before it comes to the point of discontinuing the training of a resident, it needs to be agreed upon what would be a classical situation of failure in which both the chiefs responsible for training and the residents agree that training is better discontinued. The author describes his experience with the real course of events in 7 cases he witnessed in 22 years.

Keywords: Internal standards, breach of standard, failure of residency training.

It is obvious that in the training of residents sometimes the unhappy occasion arises that the senior doctors in a training program realise that one of their residents is failing to meet the required standard. The question arises how to handle this problem and when discussing the case among the senior staff members, it soon becomes clear that the performance of the same resident is frequently judged differently by the senior staff members. This is not only due to the different personal experience, the closer or less close association of a senior doctor with that resident, but it pretty soon becomes clear that the definition of the standard is also variable among senior staff members. A discussion of the subject of this article therefore needs to start with the problem of defining the standard.

What is a Standard?

The subject of this paper are medical standards in the narrower sense, i.e. standards ruling surgical procedures or patient treatment. These medical and surgical standards require strict adherence by junior staff members. They need to be separated from the whole body of recommendations, guidelines, attitudes, modes of communication that constitute "the standard" within a department in addition to true surgical and medical rules.

Although it seems easy to elaborate a written standard concerning a certain topic, e.g. how to do a craniotomy in an acute epidural hematoma in the temporal region, it soon becomes clear that to elaborate written standards for the whole department on all matters would be a huge task. Therefore it is quite unlikely that many neurosurgical units exist in which a local standard on all questions of patient care and operative techniques are put down in writing. If they did exist, it would be of interest how the internal variation in attitudes between the senior staff members was accommodated during the writing-up of the departments' standards. The further question then arises as to how to document these standards and how to keep them up-dated during the steady flow of new facts from the literature. Other questions come up like: is everything you do in a way different from the written standard really wrong? Some junior doctors may have worked in other departments with quite different rules. Does the establishment of a written standard for every procedure and every patient condition not lend itself to be the basis for law suits? How would lawyers handle minor differences and the many unimportant variations of doctors' approaches to a given medical problem? With any attempt to define a standard a number of problems arise: Who in the department is going to define it? What about its reproducibility within the department and the many doctors involved in teaching? What about the documentation of the standard and the maintenance of that documentation? What about the independent status of the various attending neurosurgeons in the United States, the different consultants in Great Britain or of the *Oberärzte* in Germany who are entitled to have their own opinion and responsibility. How to handle the updating of a standard according to the current literature (with its often differing opinions)?

On the other side it is obvious that certain important issues need to be regulated by an obligatory common internal standard, while other issues of minor significance can be left to each doctor's discretion. Certain standards concerning vital questions are easily understood and well accepted by every member of the senior and junior staff. Thus, meaningful standards should only be defined concerning important aspects, but they should not try to regulate each detail of a doctor's life.

Hospital systems, national customs, ways of teaching can be so different from country to country that any attempt to define a standard of treatment, against which a definition of a breach of standard can be put forward, becomes problematic. The less hierarchical a hospital system is, the more liberal standards have to be defined. When I worked as a student in a department of surgery in a foreign country, I saw the consultants do operations about which the professor of surgery only shook his head sadly and made sarcastic and bitter comments. How can you develop a standard of a department if one attending neurosurgeon needs 300–600 ml of blood for a shunt during 2–3 hours of operation time, whereas another attending in the same unit needs one and a half hours and 100 ml of blood for an aneurysm.

If we have difficulties to define a standard, what then is a failure to meet a standard. Clear-cut criteria are not so difficult to describe once you restrict yourself to very basic issues. Also it should be tried to achieve an agreement both by trainees and teachers as to what constitutes a failure to meet a standard. Despite all the problems discussed before, this is much easier in daily practice. More difficult is the question of whether a failure or a violation should be documented or not. Personally, I would recommend to document and discuss it with the trainee immediately, once he violates the standards once or even frequently. As a consequence an internal report system involving all the senior staff members needs to be installed. The best way to do this would be by asking for regular evaluation sheets for each trainee from every senior staff member.

Residents' Attitudes

The opinions of the residents concerning the standard are detailed in Table 1. Staff meetings as well as written standards are both accepted by a majority of the residents. Contrary to what I expected, residents expressed to have no problems to recognize the common standard among the senior staff members. If they realize more severe differences in the management between the senior doctors, they prefer to discuss this matter in a staff meeting.

How do residents wish to handle the problem of a violation of a standard? Forty-eight percent want to discuss this among their resident colleagues, including open critique. A vast majority prefers to speak only with the relevant colleague. However, if asked specifically, 40% wish to have a senior staff member informed only if it is an important matter. No one would speak to a senior staff member if it is an unimportant matter. Only 36% wish to have the chief informed if it is important. Another 36% did not indicate that they would speak with the chief, even if it is important. What do residents think of a failing resident (Table 1)? This is a surprisingly clear attitude. They feel in a vast majority that it is acceptable to be told to change to a non-operative speciality and they want to be told by the chief in private (80%). The majority felt the appropriate time point would be after the second year or even later.

In summary, the attitude of the residents is as follows: Residents have no problems if several senior staff members have slightly different standards and the majority accepts oral communication about standards. If they notice a breach of standard by a resident colleague, they would prefer to talk openly among themselves. The vast majority prefers only to

Table 1. *Residents Survey*

- How should standards be set up?
  - 54% in written form
  - 68% staff meetings
- Can you manage to recognize the common standard among several senior staff members?
  - 72% no problem
  - 8% usually well
- If you can't – how do you want it cleared?
  - 28% written form
  - 40% staff meeting
  - 8% more uniform
  - 12% more flexible / no standard
- How to handle grave breach of standard by a resident?
  - 48% talk openly among resident colleagues
  - 16% don't talk openly
  - 12% only without critique or anonymous } 28%
- How and whom to tell?
  - 68% only to relevant colleague
  - 12% in small group
- Tell it to a senior staff member / chief?
  - 20% yes
  - 40% if important, yes } 60%
  - 4% no
  - 0% yes
  - 36% if important, yes } 36%
  - 16% no
  - 20% no reply } 36%
- Can a chief tell a resident to change to non-operative speciality?
  - 72% a chief can do it
  - 20% chief plus senior staff can
- Should he do so?
  - 80% yes, alone
  - 12% yes, plus senior staff
  - 8% no
- When should he do so?
  - <1 yr: 1   2 yrs: 7   3 yrs: 4
  - 1–2 yrs: 6   2–3 yrs: 3   4 yrs: 1

Table 2. *Examples for Repetitive Breach of Standard*

- Unprecise description of discordant findings in case of recurrent disk prolapse in X-ray conference
  - 36% discuss case + mistake
  - 36% teach again
  - 12% admonition
  - 8% warning + questioning job } 24%
  - 4% sanction
  - 4% teacher's self-critique
- Repeated failure to do clear, correct ward round on time
  - 10% discuss case + mistake
  - 40% teaching } 58%
  - 8% admonition + teaching
  - 8% admonition
  - 24% questioning job
  - 4% sanction } 36%
  - 8% no reply
  - 4% teacher's self-critique
- Repeated wrong standard trepanation
  - 24% discuss case
  - 48% teaching } 76%
  - 4% no reply
  - 8% sanction
  - 16% questioning job
  - 12% teacher's self-critique

speak to their colleague and they would only speak to senior colleagues if it is very important, whereas 36% would never speak to the chief or chose not to reply.

Breach of Standard

In the survey three situations were detailed in Table 2, described to the residents. Keeping in mind that in all three examples it was meant to be a *repetitive* breach of the standard it is somewhat surprising that 72% of residents feel that it is enough to talk about it and try to teach again. The response to a repetitive poor performance concerning a clear correct wardround on time is that 36% of the residents would react quite heavily but 50% ask only for discussion and teaching. Even in the more serious case of a repetitively wrong standard trepanation, 76% of

residents plead for talking and teaching but not for action. The responses of the residents to these examples show clearly that residents want to re-train, excercise and talk about their mistakes but they rarely accept sanctions.

The consultants' opinion concerning the three examples for repetetive breach of standard (Table 2) was also asked from 12 consultants, 10 of which answered the questions. The problem of the discordant neurological finding in the x-ray conference led 6 out of 10 to the discussion of the future in the job. The problem of the clear, correct ward round in time again brings 6 of 10 consultants to the discussion of the future in the job and the wrong standard trepanation would lead 5 to discuss the future in the job and only one of 10 to discuss, and re-train. There is a remarkable difference in the attitude comparing the people who train, compared to those who are trained. The most likely explanation for these differences seems to be that the senior staff people have come to the conclusion that a resident who has been several years in his residency and is unable to fulfill the three tasks runs a high risk of never being able to do it correctly. From my own experience I would like to add that residents tend to forget how frequently their weaknesses have been pointed out.

How to Handle the Problem of a Failing Resident

This paragraph only makes sense, if one accepts that residents can in fact fail. Once this is agreed upon, it has to be decided which frequency of significant breaches of standard constitute a severe enough substandard level that failure may happen. The obvious first step would be to notify the resident that this problem is developing. The discussion of the problems and the resulting consequences for his intensified training, his need for more support and supervision will be defined and the resident will enter a period of closer observation. The various levels of the reaction of the training staff are given in Table 3. In the author's department it has been a constant policy that all serious degrees of sanction are based on a common decision by the senior staff members.

It was confirmed in many discussions that in the process of dealing with a failing resident sanctions may be unavoidable after corrective measures, admonitions, and prolonged periods of intensified retraining have failed. As is shown in Tables 3 and 4 in the author's experience sanctions are only applied as the fourth or fifth step in a sequence of events. Contrary to what residents seem to be afraid of, sanctions do not only have negative aspects for them, but can also be understood to have positive aspects, too (Table 4). The withdrawal of the privilege to decide alone is automatically associated with an experienced colleague making the decisions and gives an opportunity to exercise decision making. Thus, sanctions do not only have penalty character but also contain elements of control, support, and supervision.

If a decision has been made that a certain resident will no longer be considered a candidate to finish his residency training, this is not automatically associated in Germany with dismissal from his job.

A very important principle of the public services disciplinary code is that it does not allow disciplinary action based on presumed or expected poor performance, only based on repetetively happened poor performance. This is difficult to understand considering the special case of a surgical resident. The situation is not made easier by the fact, that in many of the 16 Länder the university laws passed by regional parliaments force the university administrations to sign a 6-year contract with the trainees. The legal situation continues to be difficult for the unhappy case where residency training has been discontinued because of a failure to meet the standard. A certificate of employment according to the standing jurisdiction of the highest court has to follow two important rulings: Certificates of employments "... must not damage the further employment ..." and "... must not contain negative statements concerning the qualification and the performance ...".

Apart from the legal aspects there are some real experiences to be reported. The author has witnessed 7 cases in three departments in which residents were jugded by their superior to be failures and were confronted with this conclusion in senior staff meeting. Of the 7 cases, 6 residents felt insulted, started to argue, withdrew from further discussions and started secretly to look for a new job, finally ending-up in another neurosurgical unit. In only one case the resident felt insulted, started to argue and withdrew from further discussion, but returned later, listened carefully and changed his further professional life.

Table 3. *Level and Intensity of Reaction*

– Verbal correction
– Correction plus expression of dissatisfaction
– Correction plus admonition
– Correction, admonition, threat with sanction*
– Mild sanction: repeat exercise*
– Moderate sanction: discard of some duties (OP's)**
– Heavy sanction, discussion of future*
– Last sanction: end of neurosurgical career**

*senior staff discussion, **senior staff decision

Table 4. *Sanctions and Their Positive Aspects in the Handling of a Failing Resident*

• Notification of problem
• 1-n trials of correction w/wo warning
• Sanction combined with support and retraining
  1 – withdrawal of privilege to decide alone
      (automatic support by experienced colleague)
  2 – reduction in status of independence
      (in-built control + teaching)
  3 – prolongation of training
      (more chance to repeat + deepen knowledge)
  4 – reduction of OR-activity
      (give more attention + time to remaining OP's)
  5 – interruption of OR-activity
      (time to go back to the books + patient care)
  6 – cessation of OR-activity
      (we mean it – we want you to think about changing)
• Discontinuation of training

Discussion

By necessity this paper is written from a highly subjective perspective. At the same time this article reflects experiences made in three different university departments and was influenced by discussions with the members of the training committee of the Deutsche Gesellschaft für Neurochirurgie and the training committee of the EANS. From these discussions I know that the social and legal background in some countries makes it virtually impossible to terminate a residency on the grounds of incompetence, as I was told by colleagues from Scandinavia or the Netherlands. In the majority of countries it is just plain difficult to terminate a residency on grounds of incapability, but not impossible. The situation must be especially complicated in those countries where the program director is not even allowed to select his own residents, as is the case in Spain and in France. This article can certainly not give a solution that will work in all countries.

Although in several European countries it seems to be socially unacceptable to terminate a residency, the residents who answered the questionnaire in the survey obviously felt differently. Only 25 residents took part, but they came from four different departments and the answers were collected anonymously. From frequent discussions with the participants of the German and the European training courses I know that residents are well aware of the possibility that they may fail, especially concerning the operative part in the neurosurgical training. It seems therefore very important to acknowlegde the fact, that this is an accepted possibility in the mind of residents. Personally I do not agree with the opinion of B. Richling quoted on this symposium, that if something goes wrong during the training of a resident, ". . . the teachers should be asked . . .", since both sides may fail. The failure rates of the residency training reported from Great Britain and United States, and last but not least common sense confirm the majority vote in the residents survey, namely that failure in a neurosurgical residency does occur.

The part on how to handle the process of the failing resident, making sure be gets enough chances for re-training and enough support during this period, is again based on highly subjective experience. It is thus open for discussion and does not claim to be the golden standard. Each chief of a training program has to act within the framework of his national legal standards and common beliefs of his society. It is obvious that the chiefs of training programs have to be aware of their responsibility for their junior doctors who are after all adult persons with a family to care for and a life before them. On the other hand it should not be forgotten that once the residency training is finished the newly created specialist may act entirely in his own responsibility for the coming 25 or 30 years of his professional life. Consequently, it is important to establish a fair process of regular assessment of a trainee's progress and that any measures taken in case of failure be agreed upon by all senior staff members with enough time for the resident to react and to improve his performance. At the same time, it cannot be denied that failures during a residency training do occur and that the dogmatic attitude of some societies that this is automatically due to failure of the teachers is certainly not true. Any decisions made in the process of handling a failing resident have to be open for an outside assessment, ideally confirmable by other colleagues, be carried on the shoulders of all senior staff members and always be made with the welfare of the patients in mind. It is certainly unacceptable if decision-making in this respect would be ruled by political dogma or the personal opinion of one person only. It should also not be forgotten that a weak resident allowed to finish his residency despite severe repeated breaches of standard is bound to have a very unhappy professional life.

Acknowledgements

The residents and program directors who answered the questionnaire deserve credit for their help. I would also like to thank the colleagues in the Training Committee of the EANS and Deutsche Gesellschaft für Neurochirurgie for helpful discussion.

Correspondence: Prof. J. Schramm, M.D., Department of Neurosurgery, Bonn University Medical Center, Sigmund-Freud-Strasse 25, D-53105 Bonn, Federal Republic of Germany

Acta Neurochir (1997) [Suppl] 69:106–110

When Should Residents be Exposed to Research?

H.-J. Reulen

Neurosurgical Clinic, Ludwig Maximilians University, Klinikum Grosshadern, München, Federal Republic of Germany

Summary

In this paper the planning of research in a neurosurgical training program is discussed. There are good arguments to organize research rotation after one or two years of clinical exposure rather than at the beginning or the end of the program. Teacher as well as resident can prepare the rotation more carefully selecting the topic according to abilities and interests, selecting a suitable research institution, and prepare funding if necessary. The goals of a research rotation, the various categories of basic and applied research, and the length of the research period are being treated.

Keywords: Research rotation, goals of research, categories of research.

Introduction

In his presidential address at the 1994 Meeting of the AANS, Julian Hoff emphasized that the strength of this organisation is based on its devotion to research, teaching, patient care, and in the future, to socio-economics, symbolized by a four-legged stool [5]. Research is considered here to be an integral part of the training of young residents.

In 1992, Robert Ojeman [9] presented the results of a survey of 93 neurosurgical residency programs from the USA and Canada. The survey shows that all of the programs *provided* time for research *within* their 5 or 6-year residency program; however, in some programs the resident could elect a clinical rotation instead of research. The majority of the 93 programs provided research periods of at least 12 months, some had the option to lengthen the time to 18–24 months.

Obviously the majority of the program directors were of the opinion that a rotation in research is an important component in the residency, although some stated that not every resident needs a research

rotation. It is interesting that such an elective exposure to research approach is seen in the background of many, if not most successful neurosurgical leaders. Such individuals who are actually combining a successful clinical career with research are important role models for our trainees [6,8,10,12].

When Should Research Stand in the Planning of the Neurosurgical Training Program?

Should it be done at the beginning or even before starting clinical practice, should it be done after a certain time of clinical exposure or should it rather be towards the end of the program?

Probably there is no definite and generally valid answer to this question since one will find individual success stories for all three situations. However, there are convincing arguments that a research rotation should be recommended for the majority of our trainees after at least one, but not later than two or three years of clinical practice in neurosurgery [11]. It seems that in Japan research rotation is organized in a similar way [12].

I have to confess that I have changed my opinion during the last 10 years. Originally I thought that it might be good to have the research period before the beginning of clinical neurosurgery [1,2,7]. It has become more common – at least in Germany – that young colleagues, probably while waiting for acceptance to a residency, spend time in a research laboratory and often are highly recommended for good laboratory work. With time passing I had to realize that the qualities necessary to be a good scientist are not necessarily the same as those required to become a good clinician and neurosurgeon. An excellent rating in a laboratory is no guarantee that this candidate will successfully make his way in the clinic, too. Therefore we now first observe the clinical abilities and the conduct of a young candidate, and only then choose with him a suitable scientific activity. Certainly there are exceptions, for instance, someone who already has a PhD and, for some reasons, now decides to become a neurosurgeon.

The other extreme would be to organize the research period at the end of the residency program. At this stage, an intelligent resident would know his clinical interests and also have the desire to acquire the tools for a more systematic and scientific approach to some unsolved problems. However, this is exactly the time when his surgical progress and success are greatest and his interests are focused entirely on improving his surgical skills and techniques, acquiring new surgical methods, etc. Definitely, there will be a collision of interests; often this collision will be decided by economic aspects and we will lose some very gifted young colleagues.

If the resident starts with a period of clinical neurosurgery, then there are obvious advantages for both the teacher and the trainee. The arguments for the teacher are:

- The resident can be observed in his clinical and social performance, his problem-solving skills, his ability to perform under stress, his manual dexterity, his judgement, etc. The teacher can obtain an idea of his talents through observation and regular evaluation by the staff members.
- He can discuss with him his abilities and interests and find the best solution for this individual. This means they should try to define a research area which motivates the trainee for a long term and thus will lead to success!
- He has time to look for a suitable research position in this, in another department or another institution. This position should serve the interests of both, those of the resident and those of the department, if one considers eventually a continuing activity with a research project. Therefore, the selection of the topic and of the laboratory is a very important task! It is of no benefit to have the resident participating only as a technician in an ongoing project, he should be provided with the skills for independent research.
- He has time to prepare funding of a research rotation, if necessary. (In Europe we have to consider

that learning to speak and write a fluent English is an important issue and therefore research rotation often is organized in a respective laboratory.)

Vice versa, during this initial clinical period, the resident has a chance

- to examine himself whether his decision for neurosurgery as a career has been the right one. He will find out how genuine his commitment to patient management really is and pursue training with more passionate intensity.
- He learns to deal with the unusual, complex case where he sees that routine alone is not sufficient and search of literature and reading become necessary.
- He has the opportunity to observe the work of various specialists and to develop a specific interest, for instance in vascular problems, spinal problems, etc. With this background he can plan his research rotation more specifically.
- He may have an opportunity to participate in a research project.

An important requirement in such a system is that each trainee is assigned to one staff member [9,12] who takes the role of a tutor and is responsible to discuss at regular intervals the trainee's program (or problems to fulfill the requirements) and to advise him in the above described decision process. He can play a very important role in the development and the career planning of a resident. I have interviewed a number of residents and this still is a very weak point in many departments. Whether this tutor-responsibility is taken by the program director or shared among the staff members, may be decided locally.

In summary, if this initial clinical period is well used, then the success of research rotation can be enhanced by carefully selecting an appropriate research topic, and choosing a well suited laboratory which serves best the needs of the resident and the needs of the department.

The Goals of Research Rotation

What do we expect and what are the goals of such a research rotation? Most of the successful academic teachers are convinced that a research rotation, if well organized, will significantly improve the individual's rational approach to the management of

Table 1. *Goals of a Research Rotation*

- Learn to make systematic observations and documentation
- Learn to analyze and interpret the results
- Learn to critically interpret the literature
- Learn to organize the new information in a written document

- become inspired by the excitement of uncovering new knowledge
- develop independent ongoing research

Table 2. *Categories of Research in Neurosurgery* [6]

- Fundamental Neurosciences
  (blue sky research)
- Applied Clinical Research
  (transmission of basic research techniques to a clinical problem)
- Laboratory Studies simulating Clinical Diseases
  (experimental cerebral vasospasm, brain edema etc.)
- Clinical Studies of Pathophysiology of Specific Diseases
- Research related to technological Innovations and to improve Surgical Techniques
- Population – Based Studies
  (classification, natural course, outcome etc.)

patients, the critical judgement of his own work and that of reports in the literature (Table 1). George Ojeman, writing in 1985 [8] on the role of research training in a neurosurgical residency, said: "The essential features of research are making systematic observations and organizing these into hypothesis and written documents. Often, but not always, this is done in planned experiments. With this general definition, research training has a place in every neurosurgical residency program regardless of the trainee's ultimate career goals and even if they do not continue with research. For opportunities to make new observations – of unique cases, the effects of therapy, pathophysiology of neurosurgical diseases, or the function of the nervous system – will occur in every neurosurgical career".

I would suggest to add some further goals which may represent a second level. The resident should be introduced to the art of science in a way that he learns and experiences the real excitement of uncovering and describing new knowledge. Also he should come to a point where he is able to start his own research project, raise funds, and teach students and younger collegues (Table 1).

We all are aware that in our training institutions, there are residents who are planning an academic career, and others who plan to follow a practice career, although it must be stressed that many trainees at this stage of their career are unsure of their interests. With the above definitions we can offer to both groups a wide range of options according to their specific interests. The various categories of research are shown in Table 2 [6].

For those, who are motivated enough, research rotation for instance could take place in a neuroscience laboratory, with the idea to apply new techniques to a clinical problem. An actual example would be the application of molecular genetics to brain tumor therapy. Laboratory studies simulating clinical diseases, for instance on vasospasm, brain

edema, etc., are classic areas. Other options could be to offer a more clinically oriented research rotation by participating in clinical studies on pathophysiology, for instance ICP-studies in the ICU, by research related to technical innovations, for instance studies on robotics, in a microsurgical laboratory, by anatomical studies to improve surgical strategies and finally by population-based studies as, for instance, by participating in a prospective clinical trial. There is ample space for further proposals.

In many European countries, training of residents also takes place in non-academic neurosurgical departments. So far, these residents mostly do not have a fair chance of a research exposure. If such departments, as for instance in Germany, are affiliated to an academic institution, research rotation could be done in the mother institution or in cooperation with it. This would leave the possibility to later switch to an academic career. This particular issue certainly needs some more consideration.

Where to do Research Rotation

Different structures are used to organize research rotation. Some departments focus exclusively on research training in a laboratory within that department under the guidance of neurosurgical faculty members who are trained in basic or clinical research. Others prefer to send their trainees to another institution, where applied clinical research is taught (for example A. Baethmann's laboratory in Munich and many others), particularly if the department does not have appropriate conditions, and finally, a third group prefers a rotation in some areas of basic research. I fully agree with Tom Langfitt that there is not one structure that is necessarily better than others [6]. The most important point is that this time is well planned in advance in order to fulfill the expectations of both, those of the resident and those of the department. A merely obligatory year spent more or less accidentally in a laboratory, most probably will not meet those expectations and is a waste of time! It is my strong belief that we should spend more time on that individual selection of the topic and the suitable laboratory. This, however, requires that the faculty members from time to time define attractive research issues which fit in with the general frame of the research program of that department.

A successful career in a modern research university depends very much on two things: the ability to generate sustained research and the ability to develop and organize a succesful clinical program. The two areas, practice and research, regularly compete for the academic neurosurgeon's time. Therefore, when choosing the research area, there are definite advantages to combine the research topic with the individual's area of clinical interest.

An essential element in such considerations are the needs and the future plans of the department. If, for instance, a department is interested in anatomical studies to improve surgical strategies, in endocrinological studies, for instance in pituitary tumors or in their influence on growth control of meningiomas, in the pathology and prevention of cerebral vasospasm, in the molecular genetics of gliomas, in the molecular mechanisms of ischemia or the prevention of the ischemic cascade with some components, the application of modern computer technology to intraoperative localisation, or robotics, this will predominantly influence the choice and the priority or the research topic.

The Length of Research Rotation

The quality of research certainly is more important than the quantity. It has been said that any time period of less than one year of research is probably not very productive. The complexity of modern biomedical science, be it molecular genetics, immunology, endocrinology, neuronavigation, computer robotics, etc., requires a certain time to learn the respective examination techniques and acquire the background of theoretical knowledge before working on a specific problem. A lengthening of that period of 12 months may be preferable from case to case, depending on the subject. Those who plan an academic career mostly would invest more time in research, and most probably they would later form the cadre of our future academic staff. In any case, the resident should finish at least one project and also be able to continue a study project by himself.

Advanced Research Training Program

An additional option could be to support qualified candidates who have completed their neurosurgical residency and are committed to an academic career, to perform an Advanced Research Training Program. Usually this should take place in another laboratory for up to two years. This program should be organized and supported on a national level. In this context I recommend the paper of Grumbach [4]. Such candidates could form the future cadre in academic neurosurgery and form the necessary link to neuroscience.

Conclusion

The advances made by neurosurgeons in neuroscience in general and in the improvement of the management of patients in particular are extremely successful. Despite our small number we are well respected in the society, and we can be proud of it. The most important issue to maintain this strong position is the promotion of research in our speciality and the application of the fruits of that research in clinical neurosurgery.

References

1. Baethmann A, Meßmer K (1992) Stellung der klinischen Forschung in der Chirurgie: Konzept der Experimentellen Chirurgie. Chirurg BDC 31 [Suppl 1]:29–33
2. Baethman A, Meßmer K (1992) Experimentelle Chirurgie. In: Schweiberer L, Izebicki IR (eds) Akademische Chirurgie. Springer, Berlin Heidelberg New York Tokyo, pp 177–181
3. Di Rocco C (1993) The identification and the education of a pediatric neurosurgeon at an international level. Childs Nerv Syst 9:197–202
4. Grumbach MM (1990) American Pediatric Society Presidential Address. Let the walls come tumbling down. Pediatr Res 28:562–566
5. Hoff JT (1994) Toward better balance. The 1994 presidential address. J Neurosurg 81:651–655
6. Langfitt Th W (1982) Research and training in the neurosurgical sciences. J Neurosurg 57:733–738
7. Messmer K (1990) Perspektiven der Experimentellen Chirurgie. Chirurg 61:248–250

8. Ojeman GA (1985) The role of research training in a neurosurgical residency. Neurosurgery 17:138–139

9. Ojeman RG (1992) Training the neurosurgeon for the twenty-first century. Surg Neurol 37:167–174

10. Pickard JD (1995) What is neurosurgical research? Acta Neurochir 133:236–238

11. Reulen HJ, Olteanu-Nerbe V, Steiger HJ (1996) The neurosurgical clinic at the Ludwig-Maximilians-University in Munich. Neurosurgery 39:1224–1231

12. Yoshimoto T, Tominaga T (1997) Contents and structure of a training program. The Japanese proposal. Acta Neurochir (Wien) [Suppl] 69:81–83

Correspondence: Prof. H.-J. Reulen, Neurosurgical Clinic, Ludwig Maximilians University, Klinikum Grosshadern, Marchioninistrasse 15, D-81377 München, Federal Republic of Germany

Acta Neurochir (1997) [Suppl] 69:111–115
© Springer-Verlag 1997

Role of Surgical Research in the Training of Neurosurgeons

K. Meßmer and **A. Baethmann**

Institute for Surgical Research, Ludwig-Maximilians-University, Klinikum Großhadern, Munich, Federal Republic of Germany

Keywords: Neurosurgical research, objection of research training, organisation of surgical research.

Introduction

As is true for other aspects of training in neurosurgery, there is no general recipe for the role of surgical research. Nevertheless, the Institute for Surgical Research of our university offers an established program for training the young generation in this field.

Surgical Research in Germany

Surgical Research in Germany is organized in a different way as compared to many other countries. At present, we have 39 medical schools at universities, 5 of them with an independent Chair for Experimental Surgery or Surgical Research, respectively. 14 of the 39 universities in Germany have institutionalized surgical research divisions, the head of which reports to the chairman of general surgery (Table 1).

The Institute for Surgical Research at the University of Munich

We were fortunate enough to have had Prof. Walter Brendel, a physiologist by training, at an early time. Hc joined the Department of Surgery of the Ludwig-Maximilians-University of Munich in 1962 at the request of the late Prof. Rudolf Zenker. His objective was to organize Surgical Research at the highest possible academic level. Walter Brendel was a very charismatic person and, thus, a successful academic teacher. Shortly after commencement of his work in Munich he received a full professorship from the University of Munich as basis for the foundation of an independent Institute for Surgical Research. A great number of young surgeons, also neurosurgeons, were associated with Walter Brendel for a while, particularly during their first steps in science. The many accomplishments of Walter Brendel for the establishment of Surgical Research at the University of Munich were in fact the reason, why the State of Bavaria made it a point to build a new institute on the campus of the Klinikum Großhadern in 1978, which was specifically dedicated to Surgical Research. In this manner, Walter Brendel and his coworkers had the unique opportunity to plan and design a research facility according to their aspirations and needs (Table 2).

The Institute for Surgical Research in 1996

The permanent as well as transient work force of the Institute consists of *physicians*, *medical students*, and *basic scientists*, most of them employed on a full-time basis. Among others, as academic staff members we have the *"Arzt im Praktikum"* – AiP –, i.e. young colleagues in their final year of medical school prior to obtain their credentials as a physician (Approbation). Furthermore, the institute is hosting *postdocs* often coming from hospitals of the Klinikum Großhadern, who are provided with a transitory leave of absence from their unit to collaborate with us. We have also *postgraduate research fellows* from outside the Klinikum Großhadern as well as from foreign countries serving intermittently as members of our academic staff. Notwithstanding all these various curricula, the backbone of the working force of the institute are the medical students who as *research*

Table 1. *Surgical Research – Germany*

– Medical Schools	39
– Chair Exper. Surg.	5
– Sections Exper. Surg./Surg. Res.	14

Table 2. *Institute for Surgical Research (LMU Munich)*

– Founded as Exp. Unit	1962	W. Brendel
– Chair for Exp. Surgery	1969	"
– New Institute (3,000 m²)	1979	"

Table 3. *Institute for Surgical Research 1996*

– Academic Staff	12
– AiP	7
– Post docs	5
– Clin. guests	7
– Foreign Research fellows	6
– German Research fellows	2
– Doctorands (Students)	48

associates (or "*doctorands*") carry out the majority of the projects. These young colleagues are usually in their third or fourth year of medical school. They apply with us to obtain a research assignment under scientific guidance as basis for their thesis paper, which eventually is submitted to the Medical Faculty of our university to obtain a *Doctor of Medicine* degree (Table 3).

Although surgical research covers a large spectrum, the main aims may be summarized as

Improvement of perioperative treatment of patients

as defined by Francis D. Moore of the Harvard University in 1973.

As mentioned, the spectrum of our scientific activities is broad (Fig. 1). First of all, we are exploring *pathophysiological mechanisms* as an objective to improve current therapies. In other words, research activities related to this subject are supported to replace present forms of treatment by better ones, which not only are more efficient but also safe. Another objective is the *development of new methods* including the translation of basic science tools to the bedside. An important issue is the *scientific training* which is taken very seriously by the institute. This includes introduction to scientific thinking for our

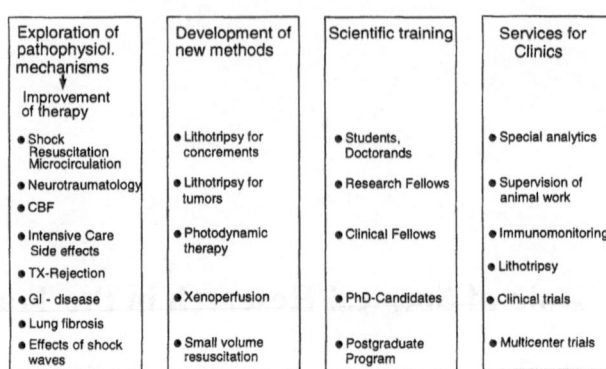

Fig. 1. Institute for Surgical Research (LMU)

students ("*doctorands*"), *research fellows* or *clinical colleagues* who are collaborating with us. Finally, the institute is providing *special services* for the hospitals on the campus of the Klinikum Großhadern and beyond. An example is allocation of *specific analytical methods*, or *supervision of animal work*. The institute has the only facilities on the campus to carry out animal experiments which, of course, requires adequate supervision. Therefore, we are offering assistance to the clinical colleagues with the preparation of applications to obtain permission for animal experiments by the Bavarian State Gouvernment. Another service is *immune monitoring* of transplant patients. Last but not least, the Institute is taking part or even supervising clinical trials in association with physicians of the various clinical departments of our medical school and outside the university.

Scope of Research

The current summary of *research activities* is given in Table 4. The Institute for Surgical Research is involved in six major research areas. One is dealing with *surgical pathophysiology* in general, another with *neurosurgical research,* which is discussed in more details below. Further areas of interest are concerned with *transplantation- and gastrointestinal-*

Table 4. *Scope of Research*

1) Surgical Pathophysiology
2) Neurosurgical Research
3) Transplantation Research
4) GI-Immunology
5) Biological effects of shock waves
6) Macrophages and lung diseases

immunology, or the *biology of shock waves*. You may know that the basic work leading to the clinical application of kidney- and gallbladder stone lithotripsy was conducted in this institute. Another program is dealing with the role of *macrophages and lung diseases*.

This wide spectrum of expertise ensures that the Institute disposes of a large array of methods and knowledge which also applies to neurosurgical research. The resulting diversity favours a climate of cross fertilization between the various scientists and groups, allowing that an advanced methodology employed in one of the teams can also be used by others.

Objectives of Research Training

It is of utmost importance to train our students in *pathophysiological thinking*. The students should be interested in pathophysiology and the exploration of pathophysiological mechanisms. Another pertinent objective is *problem recognition* in practical terms then at the bedside, to be translated into an experimental model in order to find a solution which can be taken back to the patient. In order to become an accomplished scientist who is mastering *advanced methodologies*, it is necessary to commence training as early as possible during medical education (Table 5).

Furthermore, the development of a useful *study design* and, consequently, *research protocol* is an important step for both experimental and clinical research. Other essentials to carry out a research project include expertise in *data assessment, data evaluation*, and *quality control*, finally *concise presentation of data* and *scientific writing*. The students should acquire such skills at an early point of their training, enabling them to present, discuss, and defend their own data at national or international conferences. Also, the experimental programs of our

institute offer training of surgical skills including microsurgery, which for neurosurgeons – to-be might be particularly valuable. We finally hope that the students and trainees who temporarily are associated with the Institute for Surgical Research, are forever imprinted as to maintain active contacts with academic medicine and the medical sciences.

Time Period of Surgical Research

The point addressed in Table 6 deals with the question, which time period during surgical training should be utilized for surgical research. At the Institute for Surgical Research, training starts as soon as a student of our medical school applies for a research project as "doctorand". The young colleagues are then expected to spend most of their spare time, i.e. weekends, holidays, evenings, etc. with us in the laboratory for a period of approximately two years. Another opportunity to pursue surgical research is offered to *postgraduate research fellows*. These colleagues join our institute on a full-time basis with a paid position, whereas the students of our medical school do not receive any honorarium. Obviously, they engage themselves in a scientific project by curiosity and sheer fun. Training in surgical research is also made available for *clinical residents* at a more advanced level of their academic career. These colleagues are provided with a leave of absence by their hospital for a certain period of time to join the Institute for Surgical Research on a full-time basis to carry out experimental work. However, they remain on duty in the hospital, e.g. for nightshifts or other special services. Quite often, the clinical residents are taking part in collaborative work together with the permanent staff members of the institute. Thus, collaborative projects are carried out which are designed both by the clinical partner and the permanent scientist of the Institute. Another example would be the clinical colleague who is already quite

Table 5. *Objectives of Research Training*

1) Pathophysiological thinking
2) Problem recognition (clin. → experiment)
3) Training in advanced methodology
4) Development of research protocols, study designs
5) Data assessment, evaluation, quality control
6) Presentation and scientific writing
7) Acquisition of (micro) surgical skills
8) Lifelong contact with academic medicine

Table 6. *Training – Surgical Research*

– Doctorand	Clin. student, part time, 2 years
– Research Fellow	Post doc, full time, 2–3 years
– Clin. Resident	Full time, collaborative work (Project dependent)
– PhD candidate	Full time, limited clin. obligations

advanced in his training but so far has had limited opportunities to pursue high quality research. Under these circumstances it might be difficult to make him a dedicated scientist in view of his increasing clinical responsibilities. Nevertheless, occasionally such a colleague can be successfully transformed into somebody who becomes genuinely scientifically interested. Therefore, we prefer to train clinicians in surgical research at a young age, when their mind is still inquisitive and commitment to clinical career is not exclusive yet.

Project: MD – Thesis

For scientific as well as economic reasons, the planning and execution of an experimental project for an MD-thesis should be formalized. A guideline as to how we are proceeding is shown in Table 7 as flow diagram. The first step is the *definition of the project* which is assigned to the medical student. The next step taken then by the young colleague is a comprehensive up-to-date *medline research*, followed by the development of a preliminary *experimental protocol* in collaboration with his supervisor. It is mandatory for each of our students to have a tutor during the whole period of the project until the thesis paper is concluded. Following approval of the *study design*, a *pilot study* can be initiated as basis for the final protocol. In case of animal experiments, the research protocol is submitted to the Bavarian State Government to obtain permission following its review by an ethic committee. Once the research protocol has been accepted by the administration, it cannot be changed anymore. It is only then that an animal experiment can be carried out in our institute. As a matter of fact, the students are not only in charge of running their own experiments but also of the associated procedures including laboratory methods, data assessment

Table 7. *Project: MD-Thesis*

1) Definition of project
2) Medline search
3) Protocol development
4) Protocol approval
5) Pilot studies
6) Final protocol
7) *Experiments*
8) Data evaluation
9) Research seminar
10) Presentation (congress)
11) Submission of thesis

Table 8. *Scientific Training*

1) *Seminars*
   ICF-Research Seminar
   Pathophysiology
   Methodology
   Study design
   Computerized data assessment
2) *Group conferences*
3) *Project oriented tuition*
4) *Daily supervision*

and evaluation. When the project is approaching its conclusion, the student is required to present the results or the state of the project in a formal research seminar of the Institute.

Scientific Education Program

As shown in Table 8, the *scientific education program* consists of various components. A formal *research seminar* is organized on a weekly basis. They are supplemented by ad-hoc seminars which are both program- and method-oriented, i.e. towards pathophysiology, specific methodologies, and technical issues, such as *study design* or *computerized data assessment*. In addition the various groups of this institute have their own special conferences with attendance of the scientific and technical staff and students. We provide also *project oriented tuition* and, needless to say, a more or less *daily supervision* of our younger colleagues in training by the scientific staff members.

Publications

In view of the information provided in this paper on the philosophy of the scientific training by the Institute of Surgical Research, the question arises of how

Table 9. *Institute for Surgical Research: Publications*

		1993	1994	1995
– *Original articles*				
Total		60	72	51
First author	Staff member	28	43	22
	Collaborator	24	23	26
	Stipendiate	8	6	3
– *Review articles*		14	9	3
– *Contrib. to books/proceedings*		55	43	20
– *Abstracts*		61	57	65

successful this concept is functioning, particularly as regards its scientific productivity. Table 9 gives a summary of our publications during the years 1993 to 1995. The publications are ranged according to the first author being staff member, collaborating clinician, or research fellow hosted by the Institute as "stipendiate". The figures reflect that more than fifty percent of the original articles are published not by the permanent staff members but by our scientific collaborators or research fellows hosted by the Institute. As is shown, the number of original articles or abstracts submitted per year is well balanced, indicating that the data submitted in abstracts almost always lead to publication of an original article.

Beacons of Neurosurgical Research

Concerning the point of how successfully neurosurgical research is blooming at the Institute for Surgical Research, the impressive list of scientists and clinicians as summarized in Fig. 2 needs no explaining. The accumulation of alumni shown in this table, who during a certain phase of their early career stayed with us for months or years is meanwhile covering a time span of approximately 35 years. The table does not contain those colleagues who still are associated with us. Of the altogether

Table 10. *Virtues of Surgical Research*

– Curiosity
– Methodological Expertise
– Collaborativity
– Interdisciplinarity
– Internationality
– Devotion
– Enthusiasm

forty colleagues who are named in this table, no less than seventeen have finally entered clinical neurosurgery. Of the remaining alumni, six have decided to become full-time scientists, very often in the neurosciences, which probably is attributable to their early exposure to neurosurgical research.

Virtues of Surgical Research

If one is finally asking to define the most promising virtues necessary to succeed in *Surgical Research*, the attributes shown in Table 10 appear to be particularly adequate. First of all, a drive for *curiosity* should be mentioned, then, dedication to acquire and master *methodological expertise* by conducting difficult experiments, involving microsurgery and advanced laboratory technologies. The capability to *collaborate* in a group and to carry out *interdisciplinary work* is certainly just as important. As in other areas of modern medicine, surgical research in essence is an *international* discipline requiring *devotion* and *enthusiasm*.

If a young colleague who applies for a training in neurosurgery is indeed endowed with all the attributes summarized in table 10, no doubt he will have a brilliant career.

Acknowledgements

The secretarial and technical assistance provided by H. Kleylein, E. Martin, and L. Frey is gratefully acknowledged.

Correspondence: Dr. K. Meßmer, Institute for Surgical Research, Ludwig-Maximilians-University, Klinikum Großhadern, D-81366 Munich, Federal Republic of Germany

Alumni of the Institute for Surgical Research, University of Munich 1966-1996

Prof.Dr.H.-J. Reulen, Univ. Munich	Dr.S.Vonhof, Univ. Göttingen
Prof.Dr.A..Baethmann, Univ. Munich	Dr.R.Murr, Univ. Munich
Prof.Dr.S.Prusiner, UCSF San Francisco	Dr.M.Deckert, Univ. Munich
Prof.Dr.N. Mendler, TU Munich	Dr.K. Frerichs, Harvard Univ. Boston
Prof.Dr.P. Schmiedeck, Univ. Mannheim	Dr.M.Mackert,Univ. Berlin
Prof.Dr.U.Steude, Univ. Munich	Dr.P.Temesvari, Univ. Szeged/Hungary
Prof.Dr.U.Hopt, Univ. Rostock	Dr.S.Kawamura, Univ. Akita/Japan
Prof.Dr.E. Kiffner, Karlsruhe	Dr.E.Uhl, Univ. Munich
Prof.Dr.R.Oeckler, Univ. Mannheim	Dr.S.Berger, Univ. Mainz
Prof.Dr.K.Moritake, Univ. Shimane/Japan	Dr.H.Weigt, Univ. Ulm
Prof.Dr.W.Oettinger, Trier	Dr.Ch.Abels, Univ. Regensburg
Prof.Dr.W.Lubitz, Univ. Vienna	G.-H. Schneider, Univ. Berlin
Prof.Dr.K.Maier-Hauff, Univ. Berlin	A. Rüther, Univ. Freiburg
Prof.Dr.O.Kempski, Univ. Mainz	R.Härtl, Univ. Berlin
Prof.Dr.A.Unterberg, Univ. Berlin	W. Stummer,Univ. Munich
Dr.M.Lange, Univ. Mannheim	S. Pickelmann, Univ. Munich
PD Dr.L.Schürer, Univ. Mannheim	S.Corvin, Univ.Innsbruck
Dr.C.Goetz, Univ. Munich	A.Winkler, Univ. London
PD Dr. F.Staub, Univ. Cologne	F. Spelsberg, Univ. Munich
Dr.U.v.Andrian, Harvard Univ. Boston	F.v.Rosen,Univ.Munich

Fig. 2. Beacons of Neurosurgical Research

Acta Neurochir (1997) [Suppl] 69:116–119
© Springer-Verlag 1997

Research in Neurosurgical Training: Clinical Reviews and Trials

G. M. Teasdale

Department of Neurosurgery, Institute of Neurological Sciences, Southern General Hospital, Glasgow, United Kingdom

Summary

A well prepared intellectual basis is at least as important as a sound technical training for a safe, successful Neurosurgeon. Correct decisions depend as much upon clinical information and experience as upon biomedical theory and an appreciation of the science of real life clinical research is more valuable than experience in laboratory techniques. Understanding of what makes up a good study, providing a reliable basis for clinical practice, is best gained through the training conducting personal research. The training must provide an enquiring, motivating, intellectual environment, as well as disciplined organisation and support. Successful clinical research is difficult and demanding but is one of the clearest testimonies to the quality of both trainer and trainees.

Keywords: Clinical research, clinical trials.

Introduction

Familiarity with clinical reviews and trials is a vital part in the process of life-long learning, and a basis for producing the educated, accomplished, successful Neurosurgeon. We need therefore to consider why such studies are relevant, the roles of different types of study, the factors that promote a successful experience and application and the mechanics and technicalities of performing studies.

The Basis of Neurosurgical Practice

The two vital aspects of Neurosurgery are the making of *incisions* and the taking of *decisions*. Training in the craft of surgery focuses on the production of competence in the technical skills required for safe performance of operative procedures. This can be gained through didactic teaching and apprenticeship in the operating theatre but to restrict neurosurgical education to this level is akin to producing a technical tradesman. The Neurosurgeon is elevated to the level of a professional by his responsibility for the posing and, in consultation with the patient, the taking of decisions. Questions such as "is an operation appropriate?" and, if so "what kind of operation, how should it be done, and when?" are at least as crucial in the patient's welfare as a practical per-operative procedure. Trainee Neurosurgeons need to understand how decisions are made, in particular the origin of the factors they take into consideration and the strength of evidence behind a particular approach or viewpoint.

Much of medical education in this Century has been dominated by the concepts derived from the biological approach to medicine. This reflects the immense advances in understanding the functions of the human body, the nature of disease, and the identification of increasingly specific and fundamental methods by which the body's mechanisms in both health and disease and now be influenced. Yet such knowledge essentially produces a theory of medical practice, producing the attitude, when considering a patient, that "this form of intervention *should* work". Unfortunately, concepts derived from relative purity of experimental biological investigations, whether in the laboratory or the clinic, are an imperfect basis for dealing with the vagaries and variations in both patients and diseases encountered in real clinical practice. The role of the clinical observational research, that is the basis of reviews and trials, is to enable statements such as "this treatment *does* work or more often that "this treatment is likely to work" and to be able also to put some estimate on such likelihood. To express it in the words of Osler "Medicine is a science of uncertainty and an art of probability".

What is needed in the case of an individual patient is to know the relative likelihood of a particular course of action producing a certain outcome. Although it is possible, with experience, for the individual surgeon to make an estimate based upon his personal knowledge, such experience can hardly ever be sufficiently extensive, or sufficiently precisely recalled, to form a perfect basis for practice. All too often the antidote to this is dogma. Attitudes illustrated by the saying "I am always certain about the things that are a matter of opinion" (Charlie Brown) or "I am not always right but I am never unsure" (anonymous) are surely incompatible with the faculty for ascertaining the truth that we wish to instil in the future Neurosurgeon.

The Importance of Clinical Studies

Clinical observational studies can be carried out in many ways and at many levels. These range from the report of a *single case*, of a *series of cases* – (the basis for so many neurosurgical publications) – to *case control* series (in which a group characterised by a particular outcome is identified and compared retrospectively in an effort to identify a causal factor) – to *cohort studies*, in which populations are identified prospectively and studied in parallel or series, a so called "quasi experimental design", to finally the *randomised prospective controlled trial*.

Whatever kind of clinical observational studies are carried out, the aspects that are important for the trainee are to gain an understanding of the intellectual processes involved in collection, analysis, and interpretation of clinical observations, in a systematic way. This is essential so the trainee can evaluate evidence and concepts produced from clinical experience and reports because these are the ammunition the trainee needs to enlist the support of art of probability in the battle against uncertainty. This understanding and appreciation can be gained in abstract, and there are an increasing number of publications and courses that provide education in clinical information science. Nevertheless, it is the actual doing of a clinical study that is most likely to focus the trainee's mind and to promote the awareness and understanding that is desired – provided that the experience is conducted in the appropriate way. Not all such endeavours need progress beyond presentation to a critical, informed local audience but publication of the results should be a target. The process of preparation for publication contains many hurdles from which much can be learnt. It also can provide valuable indicators and information back about the trainee, and also the training environment, and not just about "scientific" quality of mind and intellect, but about aspects of character such as common sense, enterprise, and determination. Not least important is the reality that information unpublished is knowledge lost.

The Design, Conduct, Analysis and Interpretation of Studies

The issues involved in either doing or recognising a good study are many. They include the choice of subjects, the conduct of the study, the intervention to be studied – whether prospectively or retrospectively, the choice of data both about early and the late states, and the principles of analysis and of interpretation. An appreciation of the importance of involving a statistician before the study starts is perhaps one of the most important lessons of the trainee. Statements and conclusions that are not supported by information gained are more often traced to lack of clear concepts and criticism than neglect of statistics. Indeed, lack of statistical rigour is more often shown by an over testing and an over reliance on "significance" testing.

It is unfortunately true that many published reviews and trials contain a range of defects and flaws. In this Neurosurgery is not different from all other branches of clinical medicine and specialist Neurosurgical journals are no different, in principle, from leading international general medical journals! The publication of the "CONSORT" statement by Editors of several international medical journals, containing clear and rigorous standards that must be met, is to be applauded. Editors of Neurosurgical journals should endorse similar high standards in the reporting of reviews and trials, and should promote this through the routine involvement of statisticians in the review process, recognising that this does not necessarily go with a Neurosurgical reviewer's expertise in clinical and biological matters. Good quality information on clinical studies will clearly be of ever increasing importance with the growing emphasis on "evidence based medicine". It is statutory that the group of North American Neurosurgeons, who analysed many hundreds of papers identified from Medline Search on the treatment of severe head injury, were able to discover few that meet the criteria for "class I evidence" and that even these few supported the formulation of only 4 "standards" of practice" – and that each of this was a statement against the use of an intervention!

The merits and validity of different forms of study, ranging from the case series to a randomised control trial, can be discussed but certain contrasts are undoubted. Thus, there are reciprocal relationships between ease and influence, convenience and expense. From the trainee's point of view, there are many advantages in the review of a series of cases treated previously in his unit – the data (potentially) are already available, the exercise is likely to be feasible to complete and publish within a timescale appropriate to his commitments and career development. Expenses apart from the trainee's own time, are likely to be minimal. There is no doubt that, with appropriate supervision and support, the trainee can learn much from such an experience. Unfortunately, the end result is unlikely to influence substantially the practice of the neurosurgeon himself, his colleagues, or the Neurosurgical community at large.

There can be no doubt that prospective randomised control trials provide the most influential source of information, particularly when a number of trials are combined in a "systematic review" or "metaanalysis" – even though the latter processes have their limitations. It is also necessary to recognise that large prospective randomised studies can be expensive both in time – the period from conception to publication often equalling the entire length of time currently recommended for Neurosurgical training – and financially – the cost overall being measured in millions of pounds. The meticulous amassing of immense amounts of routine information that is increasingly required in such studies can fit ill with the Neurosurgical personality and such routine data collection may be best performed by other types of staff. Nevertheless every effort should be made to involve trainees in such studies in order that they appreciate the issues involved and to provide the support and commitment needed to gain the information upon which changes in Neurosurgery will be based.

Promoting a Successful Research Experience

The successful conduct of reviews and trials reflects attributes of the trainee, his trainer and the environment. The successful trainee must have motivation and commitment, must be able to show self discipline and an ability to organise himself, others, and to harness a flow of information. There must be also an open mindedness and a willingness to learn. In order for reviews and trials of any quality to be conducted, the department concerned must have an appropriate infrastructure. The features desirable include a clear identification of the population from which the department's experience is withdrawn – without which any findings are impossible to generalise. As far as possible data collected for research purposes must be integrated with data used in routine clinical management; this promotes both the quality of information in research and its relevance of research findings to day practice. There must be due knowledgement given to the importance of the quality of data collection – be it clinical or investigative – each must be valid, consistent, reliable, routinely recorded accurately and clearly in a retrievable form. In addition, there must be an atmosphere of collaboration – within the members of the department and between departments – so that all appropriate cases can be studied and all other appropriate disciplines, skills and expertise – for example statisticians. The environment in the department must be enquiring and open minded, it must be disciplined and well ordered, it must be supportive and motivating. Trainees often ask "what should I study?" To this, I can give no better answer than that given to me at the outset of my training by the eminent British Neurologist, Prof. H. G. Miller "the best research studies arise from questions posed on a ward round". Not every trainee needs to do research, but even the most dull must recognise the many practical questions to which as yet we have no satisfactory answer.

Conclusion

The involvement of the Neurosurgical trainee in clinical research can indicate the qualities highlighted by Rovitt and referred to elsewhere in the Symposium: integrity; intelligence, capacity of work, common sense and judgement, and the faculty for ascertaining the truth. Clinical reviews and trials are the basis for the present and future clinical practices in Neurosurgery, to gain an understanding and, preferably to do such studies, is a vital component of Neurosurgical training.

References

Editorial (1996) Better reporting of randomised controlled trials: the CONSORT statement. Br Med J 313:570–571

Rovit RL (1984) Observations on the selection of neurosurgical residents. Neurosurgery 597–599

Correspondence: Prof. G. M. Teasdale, University Department of Neurosurgery, Institute of Neurological Sciences, Southern General Hospital, Glasgow G51 4TF, United Kingdom

Acta Neurochir (1997) [Suppl] 69:120–125

From the Scientific Idea to its Realisation – Principles and Strategies in Neurosurgery

R. Fahlbusch

Department of Neurosurgery, University Erlangen-Nürnberg, Erlangen, Federal Republic of Germany

Keywords: Research Foundations, project financing, realisation of research.

Our friend Douglas Miller, Edinburgh, who died all too soon, must have been a unique, highly-talented and ingenious master, in collecting grants. This was my impression when I had the opportunity to overview the list of about two dozen projects running in his department, each including money for equipment and manpower. I know from Graham Teasdale and John Pickard the considerable amount of written information that the National Health System and Medical Research Council require from a Professor in Neurosurgery when submitting grant applications.

The position of the professor and academic chairman in the UK is independent from that of the clinical chairman of the department, although both can be the same. In other systems, like in Germany, research, patient care and education are not, at present, separated. We are acting within the sensitive balance of these three poles which, in my eyes, is the key for strategical reflections, to realize a scientific idea in clinical neurosurgery. Conversely one can state, based on the Edinburgh experiences: Write a grant application and wait!

It is important and necessary to know what the reviewers are looking for. Frequently they are representatives from non-clinical disciplines or non-neurosurgical departments. You have to speak their scientific language and to convince them. I will start with general reflections about scientific ideas and their transformation to realisation and, in the second part, discuss the various forms of financial support for research.

1. Orientation Pool for Scientific Ideas

Scientific ideas are born, in general, within a pool consisting of methods, scientific societies, other disciplines, personal relationships and department facilities.

I personally believe very strongly in the fertile potential of other disciplines. We can transform their methods to neurosurgery, for example the radioimmunoassay to determine hormones and other substances from internal medicine and endocrinology. Interdisciplinary cooperation in skull base surgery is important but has no potential at all for attracting financial support – independent from this – it helps the patients and your career in surgery as a craft. Personal relationships, the influence via stimulating senior personnel, advice from experienced scientists and advertising of existing activities and projects in departments also play important roles.

True innovations are rare, for example Jannetta's neurovascular compression syndromes and Hardy's selective adenomectomy. They were born in a perspective visionary style and were already successful before the endocrinological and neurophysiological methods for physiological explanation were available.

Maturing of ideas is also rare, for example extirpation of brainstem cavernomas has been performed simultaneously in several centers in the world, because their existence could not be detected before the advent of MRI and they could be operated upon only after new knowledge became available about the anatomy and neurophysiological identification of structures in the previously untouchable area of the brainstem.

Ideas can originate from a problem or a method. One might be interested in meningiomas, or you could have experiences in in-situ-hybridisation, both with a view to bring your expertise to other disciplines, but also to a unique and fruitful combination through cooperation (Translational research).

The quality of a scientific idea is central and is characterized by its relevance (clinical consequences) to solve physiological or pathophysiological questions and its predictive potential. Is it a passing craze (medical treatment) or a long-time runner (microcirculation)? Your ideas should be fixed in a written protocol which can be the precursor of a later grant application (many times there is no vocabulary, there are no terms or no previous formulations for your problem).

How to transform the scientific idea? Shall we rely on other institutions like experimental surgery – or shall we integrate?

We have to check:

1. Which methods must be established or can already be used?
2. Which equipment exists already? Is there a laboratory or do we have to initiate a new working place?
3. Is there room for it in the department or outside?
4. Do we need an animal lab or a place for cell cultures?
5. What about manpower, how many residents, technical assistants and medical students have to be integrated?
6. What are the connections to other laboratories?
7. How can I perform the work in another laboratory?
8. What about timing? This includes the duration of the program for a grant application for two to four years and also depends on how clinical researchers can divide their time between clinical duties and pure research.

Pilot cases and pilot studies are recommended before discussing the securing financial support.

Can we use the department's research budget? Which foundation has to be taken into consideration?

Have we already contacted the local ethical committee as well as the local institution for animal research which needs in general half a year for response? There is also the waiting time for the con-firmation of your grant application. Then realisation can start.

2. Chance for Realisation

What probability has your scientific idea to be financially supported? Is it in the current frame of research guidelines? The most highly regarded projects are, from my knowledge, supported by the Deutsche Forschungsgemeinschaft (DFG), which is the most esteemed German institution for research grants, like the National Institute of Health, NIH, in USA. For the year 1995 there were 14 DFG-projects from 12 neurosurgical departments: Half of them (7) were based on molecular biological methods, 1/3 on microcirculation, brain pathophysiology, and ischemia and neuro-traumatology, 1/5 based on neurophysiological and other techniques [1]. The trend to molecular biology is similar in other disciplines, including our neighbouring fields, general surgery, ENT, neurology as well as urology. The percentage in priority programs, research units and collaborative research centers (see 3.2.2.2.) of Deutsche Forschungsgemeinschaft is with two thirds even higher.

The grants in neurosurgical research can also be reflected on international levels by the publications in the Journal of Neurosurgery, Neurosurgery, and Acta Neurochirurgica within the last $1\frac{1}{2}$ years (Fig. 1).

Spectacular developments like neurotransplantation for Parkinson's disease or microneuronal defects are not supported in Germany, because they are out of the political guidelines now. You will also

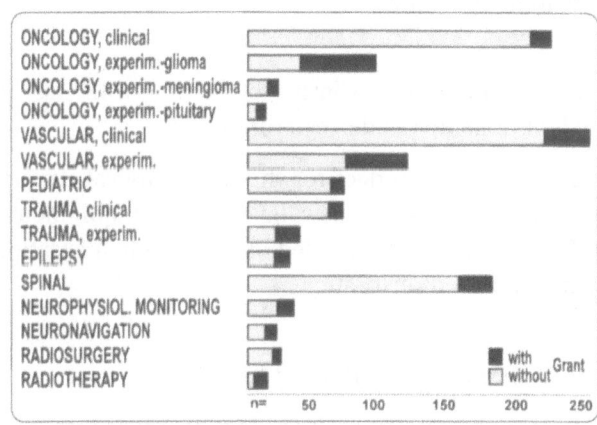

Fig. 1. Grants in neurosurgical research (from: J Neurosurg, Neurosurgery, Acta Neurochir 1/95–9/96)

miss completely neuroanatomical research and skull base projects which are necessary in neurosurgery.

3. Financial Support of Research

The institutions which support financially medical research are similar all over the world. I think that the examples listed up in the following are taken from my personal local knowledge, however incorporate general character. It can be divided into 3 levels:

1. Local
2. National
3. European

3.1. Local

3.1.1. Research Foundation of the Neurosurgical Department (Verein für Hirnforschung an der Universität Erlangen e.V.)

7 members founded this organisation. This is a non-profit making organisation of public utility which is registered at the district court (e.V.). The advantage is that no taxes have to be paid from the budget. The financial income comes from companies, private persons and patients. Scientific projects of the department can be paid by this. There is no external reviewing committee.

3.1.2. Grant Account of the University

From the financial support which is administered by the university, research projects can be paid: Mainly scholarships, research scholarships, and research fellowships.

3.1.3. University – Ministry of Culture of the Local Government (Länderregierung)

They give the budget for the neurosurgical department which allows new investments (equipment). The budget will be decided on by the administration and clinical directorate.

3.1.4. Foundations Related to University

Each university has private foundations which support research projects within the university. They can pay scholarships and equipment. In general they are regarded to be precursors of more important foundations, because their budget is limited.

In Erlangen: Marohn-Stiftung, Freifrau von Fritsch-Stiftung, Universitätsbund. The review committee consists of members of the university, they need in addition independent reviewers.

3.2. National

3.2.1. Disciplinary Foundations

3.2.1.1. In Germany: Stiftung Neurochirurgische Forschung, initiated by DGNC. They have a financial basic sum, the interests of which can be used for scientific projects. The bigger financial sums are normally paid by companies and private persons [3]. In Germany this foundation supports projects of multicenter interest within neurosurgery which will not be supported by other foundations as for example studies of general interest also in combination with technical developments by companies.

3.2.1.2. In the USA there exists a "Research Foundation – American Association of Neurological Surgeons", established in 1980. One goal is to provide a private non-governmental source of funding for research training in the field of neurosurgery. The second is to ensure the continued ability and expansion of the field of neurological surgery. The third is to demonstrate support for research endeavours by the neurosurgical community [4].

Donations for a corporate membership in this program are between US $ 5,000, – (associate) to US $ 100,000, – (associate). This includes private persons as well as families from patients and companies.

Corporate donations will be used as:

1. Research fellowships which are directed towards neurosurgeons who are preparing for academic careers as clinical investigators. This is a 2-year award, at US $ 35,000, – per year.
2. Young clinical investigator awards are given to young faculty members who are pursuing careers as clinical investigators. A 1-year award at US $ 40,000, – is provided.

The foundation's total investment in research surpassed US $ 169 million at the end of 1995.

3.2.2. Governmental Foundations

3.2.2.1. The Federal Ministry of Education, Science, Research and Technology (BMBF) supports financially medical studies of general and multidisciplinary interest, e.g. "Neuroprothesis Project": They support also a new project called "Gesundheit 2,000" in which interdisciplinary cooperation within the medical faculties is asked. They require a topic which, for example, in Erlangen is "Inflammatory Processes". The financial volume is up to half a million per year. They support furthermore 12 centers of excellence, so-called Innovations-Kollegs in the new East German Countries.

3.2.2.2. Deutsche Forschungsgemeinschaft (DFG):

– Individual Grants Program (Normalverfahren): These support research projects based on the initiative of the individual researchers. These projects are financed for a period of 3 years. A further extension is possible. The financial support is for 1 or 1.5 medical doctors, 1 or 1.5 technical assistants and disposables in general.
– Priority Programs (Schwerpunkt-Programme): The financing and coordination of the work of several researchers at different places on a certain topic or project – as a rule – for a period of up to 5 years.
– Research Units (Forscher-Gruppen): A small group of scientists who are all working on one subject (new research project at the same place, within one medical faculty). After a 5-year support, if necessary, transferred to another sponsoring institution or a different form of sponsoring, in general by the federal country.
– Collaborative Research Centers (Sonderforschungsbereiche): These are long-term research institutions of universities where scientists of various disciplines cooperate in the framework of a research program affecting interrelating fields. Neighbouring universities and research institutes can also participate in a collaborative research center. They must be acknowledged by the science council (Wissenschaftsrat).

Institutions like the National Institution of Health, United States, also support financially national projects in which non-US citizens work. This is vice-versa also possible in many other national institutions and foundations.

– Committee for Major Apparatus-Requests (Großgeräte-Ausschuß): This committee is especially powerful, because it decides about introduction of new innovative apparatus or technical systems, like the Zeiss MKM and the intraoperative MRI (if you decide for this way you have to know that research activities have to be 90% or more; these are higher evaluated than patients' care or education).

3.2.3. Others

3.2.3.1. Deutsche Krebsgesellschaft: The German Cancer Society (Deutsche Krebsgesellschaft) supports the organisation of research meetings, as subdivisions like the working group Neurooncology, and is also able to support disciplinary research studies such as the Low Grade Glioma Study (persistence is necessary; we had a ten-year long fight to be supported). This is funded by the Deutsche Krebshilfe. The Deutsche Krebshilfe supports also individual grants.

3.2.3.2. The Hannelore Kohl Stiftung supports financially projects on neurotrauma and neurorehabilitation.

3.2.3.3. Volkswagen-Stiftung: Their support is focused on topics like neuroimmunology, transplantation-immunology and robotics (Mensch-Maschine-Schnittstelle), Ganzkopf-Neuromagnetometer. The general level of funding is lower than that of DFG [7].

3.2.3.4. Deutscher Akademischer Austauschdienst (DAAD): This offers research funds for foreign neurosurgeons of younger age who want to stay 1 or 2 years to study a special scientific project in a neurosurgical department, and also for Germans who wish to stay abroad.

3.2.3.5. Humboldt-Stiftung: This supports scientific projects for 2 or 3 years for an associate professor under the age of 43 years.

3.3. European

There are scientific projects, sponsored by the European Community. They have changing scientific topics, e.g. "Biomechanical Developments", and require two or more partners in Europe.

4. Initiatives and Consequences for Chairmen

Let me conclude with initiatives and consequences for chairmen of academic neurosurgical departments. Chairmen have to develop sufficient expertise of their own, so that they can take part in the translation of the research results into clinical practise. Also they have to support research interests of residents, set up laboratories for instance for:

4.1. Clinical Biology

This could be run by PhDs in biology and biochemistry, on the pay-roll of the neurosurgical department. An adequate biological expertise has to be available as published by the EANS research committee recently [8].

Other laboratories: Multimodal monitoring, neurophysiological monitoring, image-guided surgery (influence over academic use of images, intraoperative MRI!).

4.2. Management of Research

Research has to be structured (it could be performed either as a neurosurgical research department or in close integration with the clinic). Determination of individual research time, free of clinical duties should be performed, controlled by conferences.

4.3. Intradisciplinary Cooperation (Sent to Other Departments Own Country or Abroad)

4.4. Interdisciplinary Cooperations (Neuroendocrinological and Neurooncological Working Groups; Post-graduate Seminars by DFG)

However we have to maintain our own identity within multidisciplinary teams, that means not to be only the harvestors of tissue for endocrinologists or neuropathologists.

4.5. Industry, Companies

Disorders of the CNS comprises the second largest target of the pharmaceutical market (1 billion US $

USA, 3 billions worldwide per year). Companies can be incorporated in scientific foundations [6].

We have to maintain the direction of clinical trials by neurosurgeons and not to be the harvestors of homogeneous patient groups for studies and trials for companies [2].

4.6. Medico-political relationship

The former German minister of research, Mr Riesenhuber [5], wrote 3 years ago that scientists – also neurosurgeons – should walk some hours in the forest and have a beer together with managers from the industry. A similar development of new ways of communication between scientists, managers, and politicians has been observed in the NIH, as the former neurosurgical director, Dr. Kornblith, confirmed to me some days ago. We have to understand a new way to be integrated in the market of opinion makers. They are in the medical faculty, our universities and the government. They are also in the public media (newspapers, television). Our potential integration has to be transparent.

On the other hand we should not lose the academic freedom and independency in which we are trained.

Acknowledgements

The author thanks Dr. J. Romstöck, Department of Neurosurgery, University of Erlangen, for reviewing the literature (Fig. 1), Prof G. Teasdale, Department of Neurosurgery, University of Glasgow, for advisory help, also for the manuscript, and R. Patterson, New York, for sending facts about the Research Foundation – American Association of Neurological Surgeons, presenting numerous neurosurgical colleagues who contributed in discussion.

References

1. Deutsche Forschungsgemeinschaft (1995) Jahresbericht, Bd 1
2. Pickard J (1995) What is neurosurgical research? Special Lecture EANS Research Committee Symposium. Acta Neurochir 133:236–38
3. Stiftung Neurochirurgische Forschung (1994) Mitgliederverzeichnis Deutsche Gesellschaft für Neurochirurgie, pp 40–47
4. The AANS Research Foundation. Structure and function adapted as revised by the Executive Council 11/22/91
5. Riesenhuber, Neue Produkte – neue Arbeit, Cicero Redner Preis 1995 "Die Grundlagenforschung muß aber auch wissen, daß sie den Dialog mit der Wirtschaft, die zu innovieren hat, suchen muß. Das muß in einer Vernetzung geschehen, wo der Wissenschaftler gerne mit dem Unternehmer im Wald spazieren geht oder ein Bier trinkt".

6. Tindall GT (1989) Trends in neurosurgery. The 1989 AANS presidential address. J Neurosurg 71:471–480
7. VW Stiftung (1995) Jahrbuch
8. Westphal M, Gerosa M, Fahlbusch R (1996) The role of molecular biology in neurosurgery. Meeting of the Research Committe of the EANS in Hamburg, March 3–5, 1995. Acta Neurochir 138:770–75

Correspondence: Prof Dr. J. Fahlbusch, Department of Neurosurgery, Kopfklinikum, Universität Erlangen-Nürnberg, Schwabachanlage 6, D-91054 Erlangen, Federal Republic of Germany

Acta Neurochir (1997) [Suppl] 69:126–129

Subspeciality Training in Neurosurgery

Ch. Ostertag

Stereotaktische Neurochirurgie, Neurozentrum, Freiburg, Federal Republic of Germany

Summary

Evolution for neurosurgeons is not at a standstill. The environment, competition from neighbouring fields, advances in biology and changes in the level of information available to our patients, the "market" will favour and demand subspecialisation. Subspecialists are characterized by recognized records of excellence. The best suited to impart knowledge to a clinical fellow is the senior subspecialist who is working within a group of other complementary subspecialists. To develop subspecialty expertise takes a minimum of one, preferably two years of training. Neurosurgery will retain and regain its strength as a discipline by diversification, not by clinging to monolithic uniformity.

Keywords: Neurosurgery, professional training, subspecialisation, practice standards.

Introduction

Neurosurgeons are a particular species in terms of evolutionary science. These finches of surgery thrived and vigorously grew in the environment of neurology. The principle of natural selection has favoured these finches. However, even within the species finch there is considerate subspecialisation. Some finches are living on kernels, other on insects as their beaks tell (Fig. 1). Selection is based on a set of rules, which govern variation within a species. This contains the aimless production of a spectrum of variants, the stabilisation of a selective advantage, but also the extinction of a population with defects [3].

Do we need Subspecialists?

In the process of evolution neurosurgery became a specialized branch of surgery. Historically branching of a subspeciality has always been a difficult process. Many of the readers may be familiar with the fric-

tions between Cushing and Halstedt at Johns-Hopkins or between Tönnis and the surgical establishment, respectively, when they branched off. Nowadays the subspeciality neurosurgery itself is branching, others complain and say: disintegrating. Is it branching or disintegrating, because neurosurgeons were inappropriately educated or because they find themselves in a rapidly changing and increasingly unfavourable environment?

Some interesting "environmental" aspects stand out and need to be addressed:

1. By its nature neurosurgery has always had the broadest interface with other specialities. To name a few: radiology, orthopedics, anesthesia, ENT, oncology, pediatrics, radiation therapy. When we carefully look around us we see that neurosurgery indeed is disintegrating, is loosing territories to the interfacing disciplines: Spinal territory to the orthopedics, skull base territory to otolaryngology, tumor neurosurgery to radiation oncology, vascular neurosurgery to endovascular radiology, peripheral nerve neurosurgery to plastic surgeons (Table 1).

   Why this? Because someone from a neighbouring field focused his interest and his skills on a particular problem and – as time goes by – does perform better. The only way to regain the lost territories is subspecialisation, i.e. we as neurosurgeons must do better than our competitors from orthopedics, from ENT, from plastic surgery and from radiology.

2. Another aspect introduced by Cohadon [2] focuses on our craft itself. Classically we understand an operation as a mechanical manipulation of a

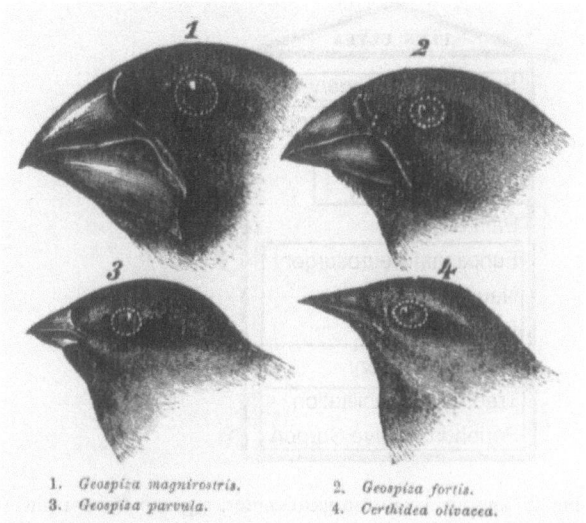

Fig. 1. Darwin's finches [3]

Table 1. *Disputed Territories*

Spinal Neurosurgery – Orthopedic Surgeons
Skull base Surgery – Otolaryngology, Ophthalmology
Tumor Surgery – Radiation Oncology
Vascular Neurosurgery – Endovascular Radiology
Periphal Nerve Surgery – Plastic Surgery
+++

localized target. However, the recent progress tends to look at the problems of illness along biological lines. Although our subject remains neurosurgical the tools become biochemical, immunological or pharmacological when needed ("molecular neurosurgery", Martuzza) [5]. A sophisticated biological knowledge is transforming the aims and the means of the traditional neurosurgical approach. Various biological techniques are likely to compete directly with classical, i.e. with mechanical neurosurgical procedures. Natural selection will favour those who can make use of the new biological knowledge and technical progress.

3. Not only medicine is changing fundamentally but also the social environment. The modern social environment favours health care as an industry. Our patients, the consumers, have become well-informed and conscious of developments in medicine. Both consumers and payers are carefully watching: What is the benefit for the patient? What does it cost? Payers and consumers ask for standards based on sound statistical evidence.

Good standards, sound statistics of efficacy, morbidity, mortality and cost effectiveness, however, can only be produced by the subspecialist. Namely the subspecialist who concentrates his work on a restricted area, and who does certain procedures with a daily routine. It has become impossible for a single individual to keep pace with all the advances and adapt to all the techniques of neurosurgery [7]. Textbooks of neurosurgery nowadays are organized as multiauthored books. In the case of the three volume textbook edited by Wilkins and Rengachary it took 428 contributors. It is unlikely that today one single neurosurgeon can fulfill all the requirements of neurosurgery with sufficient expertise.

4. Given a particular problem of a patient, both the specialist and the non-specialist have been blamed to be one-sided: The specialist knowing and applying only the specialist methods. Likewise the non-specialist, the omnipotent single hero of neurosurgery who never refers a patient to a subspecialist, often tries his own inappropriate methods on the patient's life and well-being. Both are stretching their capabilities to the extreme limits. The law in Germany requires that only board certified neurosurgeons carry out an operation. However, is case of a lawsuit also the experience of the surgeon is questioned. Could the patient have been operated on successfully by another more experienced, i.e. subspecialized neurosurgeon in another faculty?

There are still too many neurosurgeons who completed their training of the basic aspects of neurosurgery and who are not prepared or dare not devote their professional life to a limited sector of neurosurgery. However, with discipline they could excel in this limited field and improve their status. Thus subspecialisation not only presents several advantages. In the given professional, social and legal situation it seems more a necessity than a choice. What kind of problems will be left for the non-specialized neurosurgeon given the fact that our patients have booklets in hand specifying "The 500 Best", or they simply go into the Internet? Only as long as there is "asymetric information" to our consumers as to the quality of the individual worker in the field the present system can survive. Is more subspecialisation an inevitable fate? My answer is: probably yes.

Table 2. *Self-Designated Subspecialty Interest*

Spinal Surgery	36.6%
Neurosurgical Oncology	4.6%
Pediatric	30.9%
Stereotactic/Brain Tumors	3.4%
Pain/Trauma	2.9%
Cerebrovascular	12.6%
Epilepsy	1.7%
Skull Base	4.6%
Peripheral Nerve	1.7%

Source: Practice Survey. AANS Bulletin, Summer 1996

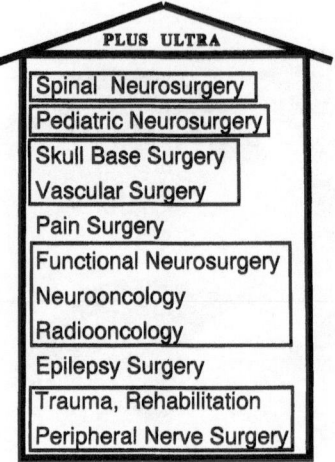

Fig. 2. The ideal neurosurgical center: a group (5+ persons) of subspecialists with complementary fields of interest provides the best training conditions for subspecialization

What Sort of Subspecialists?

A recent practice survey carried out by the AANS revealed a self-designated subspeciality interest in spinal surgery (36.6%) and pediatric neurosurgery (30.9%) among a variety of other subspecialities [1]. The "market" has already produced a fair number of recognized subspecialities. Established neurosurgical subspecialities are pediatric neurosurgery, spine, skull base, cerebro-vascular and functional neuro-surgery (Table 2). Many of them are organized as sections or even on a departmental level. Subspeci-alities such as epilepsy surgery, pain treatment, radiooncology, rehabilitation etc, are the particular focus of interest and of engaged individuals. Stereo-taxy here is not listed as a subspeciality. Stereotaxy like microsurgery is rather considered as an approach, a methodology which can be used for, and pervades now most fields of neurosurgery.

What Characterizes the Subspecialist?

Being a subspecialist and counting the thumbs of my hands I certainly do not have more than anybody else. It is not the number of thumbs but the recog-nized record of excellence which makes a sub-specialist. "When confronted with a problem he is not familiar with, the neurosurgeon is obliged to use consultants and other health care providers *with rec-ognized records of excellence as a source of informa-tion* concerning current therapies and prognoses" [4]. This admonitory statement not only applies to the field of birth defects, it applies to all fields of neurosurgery. The records are scientific statements and numbers, namely sound statistics. Nobody can claim to be a subspecialist without providing num-bers regarding cases, outcomes, mortality, morbidity, the costs and potential benefits and risks for the pa-tients, the family, the society.

The natural environment for the subspecialist where he thrives best is certainly the academic set-ting of a university, the center of excellence. As de-scribed by G. F. Rossi [6] a group of subspecialists with complementary fields of interest offers the best working conditions in terms of knowledge, efficiency and cost-effectiveness. Daily discussions and views from different angles are a prerequisite for good neurosurgical practice (Fig. 2).

How to Produce the Subspecialist?

Subspeciality training in Europe is largely undefined, unorganized and uncontrolled. How to acquire subspecialisation, where and when? Without doubt, subspecialisation is built on a good basic neuro-surgical training. Clinical fellowships are designed for individuals who have already completed their pri-mary neurosurgical training. This for me is not a point of debate. A well trained resident during his rotation has already had contact with all subspeciali-ties. After board certification he/she may realize that he/she will never become as omnipotent as neuro-surgeons were twenty years ago.

One cannot become a subspecialist during a brief visit in one or several particular units, by participat-ing in a hands-on course or in a workshop. It is not mere technical training how to perform, for example a pallidotomy. It is more than the mere exposure to a great number of standardized operations. Subspeci-ality training contains outpatient clinics and the op-portunity to carry out at least retrospective studies, i.e. publishing clinical data which will provide visibility as a subspecialist. Clinical fellowship should offer the possibility to perform basic research in a particular field. To develop subspeciality expertise takes a minimum of one year, preferably two years. Experiences with clinical fellowships issued by the European Society for Stereotactic and Functional Neurosurgery have shown that three-month fellowships are good for an evaluation period, both for the fellow and the teacher. They are, however, too short for a sufficient subspeciality training.

The best suited to impart knowledge, to educate a clinical fellow, certainly is the senior subspecialist, who works in a group at a center of excellence. It is only there that the atmosphere of questioning, criticism and accumulated expertise can be provided. Only the group of complementary subspecialists can impart knowledge of the area of special interest in a balanced way. Anyone working in isolation is not best suited to educate a clinical fellow. After subspeciality training, the fellow usually remains in continuous close contact with his instructor, which at the beginning of his practice is a safeguard and a lifeline.

References

1. Anonymus (1996) Comprehensive practice survey. AANS Bulletin, summer 1996
2. Cohadon F (1981) The future of neurosurgery. Acta Neurochir 55:169–179
3. Darwin C (1962) The origin of Species. Crowell-Collier Publ Comp, Toronto, Ontario
4. Guide to the American Association of Neurological Surgeons (1993) Position Statements
5. Martuzza RL (1992) Molecular neurosurgery for glial and neuronal disorders. Stereotact Funct Neurosurg 59:92–99
6. Rossi GF (1988) Subspecialisation in neurosurgery. Acta Neurochir 94:1–9
7. Wilkins RH, Rengachary SS (1985) Preface. Neurosurgery. McGraw-Hill, New York

Correspondence: Prof. Dr. Ch. Ostertag, Abteilung Stereotaktische Neurochirurgie, Neurozentrum, Breisacher Strasse 64, D-79106 Freiburg, Federal Republic of Germany

Acta Neurochir (1997) [Suppl] 69:130–134
© Springer-Verlag 1997

Neurosurgical Spine Fellowships: The Phoenix Model

V. K. H. Sonntag

Division of Neurological Surgery, Barrow Neurological Institute, St. Joseph's Hospital and Medical Center, Phoenix, Arizona, U.S.A.

Keywords: Subspeciality training, spine fellowship.

Introduction

Typically, a fellowship in the United States is defined as 1 to 2 years of extra training in a special interest area after a residency has been completed. The fellowship should not fulfill an area of training that was not covered in the residency. Rather, it expands upon the experience obtained in the residency and develops a specialist and/or leader in the particular area of interest. Historically, as medicine has become more complicated and sophisticated, almost by definition, it has become increasingly specialized. Therefore, the natural evolution has been toward subspecialty fellowships. With that in mind, spine fellowships in neurosurgery have been developed throughout the United States over the last several years.

The rationale for the existence of spine fellowships in neurosurgery are as follows. First, a fellowship emphasizes neurosurgeons' commitment to spine. Neurosurgery, by definition, is a specialty that treats disorders of the central nervous system, the peripheral nervous system, and its support structures. Consequently, the existence of the neurosurgical spine fellowship emphasizes neurosurgical interest in the spine in a given training program, institution, and community. A fellowship also emphasizes neurosurgeons' commitment to the spine on a national level as well – not only within their own professional organization but also in relationship with other specialities such as orthopedic surgery, physical medicine and rehabilitation, and neurology. Neurosurgery also needs superspecialists, that is, leaders in spine, and the spine fellowship is certainly

an avenue to achieve that goal. Neurosurgery also needs to be competitive for the specialty to remain vital as it is being challenged, not only in spine but also in peripheral nerve, vascular disease, and skull base, by multiple other specialties. To remain on the "cutting edge", neursourgery needs superspecialists who will become leaders in their respective specialties. Obviously, a spine fellowship will lead to a spine specialist who in turn can teach complex spine cases to residents, fellows, and medical students.

A neurosurgical resident should be trained to be a complete neurosurgeon who can handle the full spectrum of neurosurgical problems from intracranial aneurysms to thoracic lumbar instrumentation. It is, however, inconceivable that an individual will become an expert or specialist in all of these techniques. Consequently, spine fellowships exist to build upon the experience obtained by the residents during their training years.

There are also several disadvantages associated with a neurosurgical spine fellowship. Unless an institution's surgical volume is adequate, spine fellows compete with residents for cases and, hence, for training. The fellowship adds 1 to 2 years to an already long neurosurgical training program. The spine fellowship emphasizes specialization, which could contribute to the fragmentation of neurosurgery. Also, in some training programs, individuals may be so well trained in spine that they are already specialists in spine, but they might lack credibility because they have not done a fellowship. The existence of a fellowship also fuels the controversy of whether certification and or accreditation should be required.

Criteria for a Neurosurgical Spine Fellowship

Institutions sponsoring neurosurgical spine fellowships should have an Accreditation Council for Graduate Medical Education (ACGME) accredited residency in neurological surgery. The program should have a close relationship with orthopedic surgery and should maintain a collegial relationship with related clinical specialties, including but not limited to physical medicine and rehabilitation, neurology, radiology, pathology, laboratory medicine, anesthesiology, and medicine. Modern facilities and equipment to support the overall education program must be readily available and functioning. Such facilities consist of an outpatient/inpatient clinic, up-to-date imaging facilities, and resources for laboratory, rehabilitation, and research. The operating room must be state-of-the-art and house modern equipment for surgery of the spine. The director of the fellowship must be certified by the American Board of Neurological Surgery or possess equivalent qualifications and have a specialized interest in spine and is recognized as such. There must be a sufficient number of program teaching staff with the diversity of practice to support a broadly based educational experience for all fellows. The fellowship director and teaching staff must exhibit an ongoing commitment to the educational program; be engaged in research activities and other scholar activities; and clearly demonstrate high ethical, humanistic, and professional standards in the care of their patients.

The spine fellowship must not interfere with the training of residents in the treatment of spinal disorder. Therefore, the host institution must have a large number and variety of cases to fulfill the needs of both residents and fellows. Each individual fellow should be exposed to at least 25 thoracic lumbar instrumentations a year. Neuronal and biomechanical research should be part of the fellowship. Besides inpatient care, a follow-up outpatient clinic should also be part of the training. The fellows should be responsible for regularly scheduled neurosurgical consultation, and clinical and laboratory research projects should be assigned to fellows in conjunction with faculty supervision. Spine neurosurgical fellowships in the United States do not have a separate certificate of added qualification but are indirectly monitored by the Neurosurgical Resident Review Committee (NRRC). If the NRRC determines that the training of the resident is impaired because of the presence of a spine fellowship, it can deny certification of the residency program unless the fellowship is downsized or curtailed.

The candidate applying for fellowship must have completed an approved neurosurgical residency program and have passed the written examination of the American Board of Neurological Surgeons or be board certified (or equivalent). At present, there is a matching program in neurosurgical fellowships in the United States but participation by the institution and the applicant is voluntary.

Guidelines

In 1991, a guideline for neurosurgical spine fellows was developed in the United States under the auspices of the Senior Society of Neurological Surgeons (see Appendix). These guidelines were endorsed by the Congress of Neurological Surgeons (CNS), by the American Association of Neurological Surgeons (AANS), by the then existing Spine Task Force, and by the Joint Section of Disorders of the Spine and Peripheral Nerves. The guidelines detail the educational program, facilities and resources, and the special knowledge and skills that an individual fellow will develop during the fellowship. These guidelines were sent to all program directors. The guidelines were not officially endorsed by the NRRC, but as mentioned, the NRRC has indirect control of the fellowship by ensuring that the fellowship does not dilute the training of residents.

In 1991, the Joint Section of Spine and Peripheral Nerves also voiced support for the existence of neurosurgical spine fellowships by stating that they should exist to develop the spine specialist, to stimulate research in spine, to produce leaders in spine, and to improve the spine training of residents as long as the spine fellow does not compete with residents.

The Phoenix Model

The Neurosurgical Spine Fellowship in Phoenix, Arizona was started in 1988 at the Barrow Neurological Institute. Twelve fully trained fellows have finished the program and two are presently in training. Of the 12 fellows, six have full-time appointments in academic programs ranging from professor to assistant professor and three have part-time academic appointments. In 1992, the fellows formed a society (Sonntag Spine Society), which has an annual scientific meeting and meets the day before the annual meeting of the Joint Section of Disorders of Spine and Peripheral Nerves.

The two fellows at the Barrow Neurological Institute rotate service, dedicating 6 months to clinical service and 6 months to the laboratory. Research performed in the laboratory ranges from neuronal research to biomechanical research, the latter under the direction of Dr. Curtis Dickman and Neil Crawford, Ph.D., a specialist in biomechanics. In the clinical service, the fellow acts as a junior attending. He is a teacher and tutor for residents and acts as the fellowship director's right-hand man. The fellow does have some weekend call. Fellows are expected to conduct and/or present at weekly rounds and to publish articles in both the clinical and laboratory arenas. Fellows on the 6-month clinical rotation are expected to participate in all major spine surgeries as either the primary surgeon or the assistant and, of course, as a teacher. Daily patient rounds with the attending and the house staff are mandatory. Fellows are also expected to participate in the outpatient clinic, which is vital in the appropriate care of an individual with spinal disorder.

As mentioned, it is extremely important that the spine fellow does not interfere with the training of residents. This condition primarily depends on surgical volume. Fortunately at the Barrow Neurological Institute, the surgical volume is high. For example, from October 1994 to October 1995, the total number of neurosurgical procedures was 4,071. The total number of spine procedures was 863, and the total number of spine procedures with instrumentation was 247. In 1995, the residents at the Barrow Neurological Institute were surveyed to determine the advantages and disadvantages of a spine fellowship. According to the residents, there were several advantages. (1) Spine fellows act as tutors. (2) The fellowship emphasizes spine. (3) Spine fellows are helpful adjuncts at conferences and in the operating room. (4) Spine fellows were perceived as "on the whole a very positive influence." According to the residents, the only disadvantage was that a spine fellow might compete with the residents for cases, but most found no associated disadvantage at all.

Conclusion

Spine fellowships are important for the very existence of neurosurgery, emphasizing neurosurgery's commitment to the spine and will keep neurosurgery competitive with other specialties. Spine fellowships should be restricted to institutions with enough surgical volume to avoid diluting the residents' training. The Fellowship should train individuals who have successfully finished their neurosurgical training, to become leaders in Spinal Surgery and most importantly, to improve the care of patients who are suffering from some spinal disorders through clinical and basic research.

Appendix

The guidelines were developed by the Spine Task Force (chairman D. Velly), appointed by the AANS and Society of Neurological Surgeons.

Guidelines for Spinal Training for Neurosurgical Residents

I. Educational Program

A neurosurgical resident training program should include the listed requirements, which should result in a neurosurgeon who is a complete spinal surgeon. Training in neurological spine surgery should include in-depth study, prevention, and treatment of spinal column diseases, disorders, and injuries by medical, physical and surgical methods. The program must have regularly scheduled subspecialty conferences with active faculty participation in conjunction with other disciplines included in treatment of spinal disorders, such as radiology, physical medicine, etc. The program must emphasize the diagnosis of clinical disorders of the spine, the pathogenesis of these disorders, the operative and non-operative treatment modalities available in managing these disorders, and the results of complications of such treatment. Fellowships are only needed for those individuals who want to intensify their interest and specialize with training over and above the complete spinal training in the residency.

II. Facilities and Resources

Modern facilities and equipment to support the overall educational program must be readily available and functioning. These include out-patient, in-patient, imaging, laboratory, rehabilitation, and research resources. Operating rooms must be state of the art and contain modern equipment for surgery of the spine. The program director must be certified by the American Board of Neurological Surgery or possess equivalent qualifications. There must be a sufficient number of program teaching staff with a diversity of backgrounds to support a broadly based educational experience for all residents. The program director and teaching staff must exhibit ongoing commitment to the educational program in research and other scholarly activities, and clearly demonstrate high ethical, humanistic, and professional standards in the care of their patients.

III. Special Knowledge and Skills

– A. Basic Sciences
    1. Anatomy:
        a. Spine and Joints
        b. Occipital-cervical junction
        c. Cord, including detailed anatomy of the spinal cord, its covering and vascular supply
        d. Nerves
            1) Dorsal root
            2) Ventral root
            3) Ganglion and sympathetic chain
            4) Lumbar and brachial plexus
            5) Histology
    2. Spinal Cord Physiology:
        a. Cellular neurophysiology
        b. Cellular biochemistry
        c. Treatment options to treat normal/abnormal cellular physiology or cellar biochemistry
    3. Biomechanics:
        a. Various theories concerning the stability of the spine, the normal motion, the abnormal motion, and how the normal motion becomes an abnormal motion by the various surgical interventions and various pathologies.
        b. Fracture classifications
    4. Radiology:
        a. MRI
        b. CT
        c. Myelogram
        d. X-ray

– B. Clinical
    1. Perform:
        a. Examinations:
            1) Neurological
            2) Mechanical
            3) Muscular
        b. Procedures:
            1) Myelograms
            2) Lumbar punctures
            3) C2 punctures
    2. Be Able to Treat/Understand/Do:
        a. Back/neck pain
            1) Acute
            2) Chronic
            3) Compensatory
            4) Degenerative
            5) Infectious
            6) Traumatic
        b. Degenerative disease: Surgical
            1) All levels of spine
            2) Anterior/posterior approach
            3) Diskectomy
            4) Foramenotomy
            5) Corpectomy
            6) Laminectomy
        c. Neoplasms: Surgical
            1) All levels of the spine
            2) Anterior
            3) Posterior
            4) Corpectomy
            5) Laminectomy
            6) Tumor biology
            7) Epidural
            8) Intradural
            9) Intramedullary
        d. Trauma: Non-surgical
            1) Traction
            2) Halo application
            3) Tong application
            4) Halo-vest application
            5) Orthotics to all parts of the spine
            6) Reduction techniques
        e. Trauma: Surgical
            1) All levels of the spine anterior and posterior approaches
            2) Corpectomy
            3) Laminectomy
            4) Foramenotomy
        f. Congenital Processes
            1) Tethered cord

2) Rachischitic defects

g. Infectious Processes

3. Be Able to Understand:
   a. Fusion Principle
      1) Biology of bone
      2) Biomechanics of fusion
   b. Neurophysiologic Monitoring
      1) EMG – Nerve conduction
      2) SSEP-MEP
      3) Intraoperative nerve monitoring
   c. Peripheral nerve injury

4. Be Able to Do:
   a. Anterior Approach
      1) Transcervical
      2) Transthoracic*
      3) Transabdominal*
      4) Retroperitoneal*
   b. Posterior Approach
      1) Laminectomy
      2) Far lateral to occipital-cervical junction
      3) Extra cavity
      4) Costotransversectomy
      5) Transpedicular
   c. Fusion techniques – Anterior
      1) Anterior cervical
         a) Interbody
         b) Plating
         c) Strut crafting
      2) Anterior thoracic/thoracic-lumbar/lumbar
         a) Instrumentation
         b) Strut crafting
         c) Methylmethacylate
         d) Combination
   d. Fusion techniques – Posterior
      1) Occipital Atlas Axis
         a) Bone grafting
         b) Instrumentation
         c) Methylmethacylate
      2) Cervical-subaxial
         a) Bone grafting
         b) Instrumentation
         c) Methylmethacylate
      3) Thoracic/thoracic-lumbar/lumbar
         a) Instrumentation
         b) Pedicle fixation
         c) Methylmethacylate

IV. Ideal Spinal Training for the Neurosurgery Resident

A. Neurosurgery faculty identified with principle professional interest in spinal surgery.
B. Six to twelve months in laboratory with experience in biomechanics/neuronal research.
C. Separate clinical teams for spine with dedicated full-time supervision.
D. Biomechanic and bioengineering departments readily available.
E. Orthopedic Department active collaboration
F. Physiatry/Rehab Department
G. Psychiatry Department
H. Neurology Department
I. Developmental Biology
J. Spine Outpatient Clinic
K. Pediatric Spine Specialist

Correspondence: V. K. H. Sonntag, M.D., c/o Neuroscience Publications, Barrow Neurological Institute, 350 West Thomas Road, Phoenix, AZ 85013-4496, U.S.A.

---

* Other surgeons may do the opening

Acta Neurochir (1997) [Suppl] 69:135–139

A Model Fellowship in Pediatric Neurosurgery

A. J. Raimondi

Pediatric Neurosurgery, University of Rome "La Sapienza", Rome, Italy

Keywords: Subspeciality training, pediatric neurosurgery.

Introduction

I should begin this essay in a collegial manner, for we are – all of us – colleagues, and many of us have been colleagues for many years. But more, we have been gathered by one of the foremost leaders in academic Neurosurgery, and in Education within our general speciality and its many aspects, Hans Reulen, to review and to renew our thinking. Let's rethink this entire matter . . . at truly international levels.

Regarding my title and the message I shall convey, I wish to state in straight forward a manner as possible that the problems we face must be identified immediately and stated clearly: "Does the formal recognition of pediatric Neurosurgery (or any other discipline) as a sub-speciality exclude general neurosurgeons from working in these areas?" The model program I propose, and its philosophical underpinnings say. . . . "NO!". However, there are two factors which must be recognized: Reality and Price.

One must first establish the parameters within which such a title may have a meaning, or be of value to the consumer. At the same level, it is essential to clarify the individual components of this noun phrase – pediatric. . . . Neurosurgery – with regard to organizational participation, structural composition, accreditation, and the legal implications of their activities, on the one hand, and which their existence imposes upon Neurosurgery, on the other. I shall speak only about the implications of a Model Pediatric Neurosurgery Fellowship . . . not about Pediatric Neurosurgery Units.

It is the interaction between organized Neurosurgery – especially that in the USA – and the "extraparlamentari" which complicate matters to no small amount! ("Extraparlamentari" is an Italian term for those who have no official jurisdictional or representative office, but who organize pseudo-legal groups.) Since we must provide University/Teaching-Hospital programs and patient care in the sub-speciality of Pediatric Neurosurgery, we must recognize that children have particular anatomo-pathological problems which require particular Neurosurgical techniques . . . and facilities.

It is our responsibility to unravel these hardened positions, skewed perspectives, and to look simply upon the reality which is that pediatric Neurosurgery is a sub-specialty and that Neurosurgery* must provide for its educational, academic, and professional needs, within the structure and function of Neurosurgery. It serves no purpose to discuss structural realities with such artificial terms as "focused training" [1] for "sub-specialty training" and "evaluation" for "accreditation". They are linguistically and semantically incorrect, coined only to find a path which belongs neither to the suppliants nor the accrediting bodies.

We cannot solve a problem with euphemisms. We must look at its elements realistically, and realistically we must concede that science, and its applied arts, are constantly in change. As these activities change we change with them. In this sense, this conference is most timely: it permits us to accept the advances in our profession by structuring them into

---

* In this text Neurosurgery is capitalized (N) since it is used as a personification of an abstraction, giving it the attributes of a person

teaching programs which are to be conceived, organized, and conducted by Neurosurgery, not leaving the present and future subspecialties to do this independently. The perspective of a subspecialist suffers a blind-spot which may be metaphorically described as the mirror image of that of a generalist. They must work out together, difficult and challenging though it may be, the programs and the teachers. One group or the other will delegate the responsibility to a limited number of people who may be vulnerable to personal interests. The very success of the EANS (until now), the AANS, and the CNS teaching courses speak eloquently of the validity of this thesis! [2]

Elements, Composition and Conduction of a Model Fellowship

With this introduction, I should like to present first and discuss subsequently the 1. elements, 2. composition, and 3. conduction of a *Model Fellowship* in Pediatric Neurosurgery. In preparing this essay, I have drawn upon my own experiences and writings [3,4,5], and upon those of Jean Francois Hirsch (the leading pediatric neurosurgical academician in the Eastern Hemisphere) [6].

I. Elements

These consist of population base, a children's hospital, administrative independence, and a separate budget.

A. Population Base

It is a fact that in the cities of Chicago (2,500,000 inhabitants) and Paris (2,160,000) there are approximately 0.06 Neurosurgery beds per 1,000 inhabitants, the ratio of pediatric to adult Neurosurgery beds being 1:10. Therefore, the ratio of pediatric Neurosurgery beds to population is 0.006:1,000. In Paris at the present time these are all zoned into one center, L'Hôpital des Enfants Malades. In the Chicago Metropolitan Area there are four centers, with a fifth in the last stages of planning. (I personally prefer the Chicago choice, for centralization has very real geographic and human disadvantages: transportation problems for the majority of families, an absence of inter-institutional competition). Paris has a metropolitan (cathement) population of 10,000,000, Chicago of 6,500,000.

B. Children's Hospitals

Most people would agree that the most cogent arguments for the sub-speciality of pediatric Neurosurgery have to do with the particular anatomical, epidemiological, and sociological characteristics of children, on the one hand, and the necessity of immediate availability of other pediatric sub-specialists, on the other hand. In a children's hospital one has a physical setting designed and built for children, providing professionals of all medical and paramedical categories (from other sub-specialists and nurses through paramedical to administrative and teaching) to confront their problems. Hence, the pediatric neurosurgeon is supported by other specialists, social workers, psychologists, etc., etc. The child and the families are in a children's world. Everyone is comfortable with children and parents. These points, once mentioned, are so intuitive as to render explanations tedious.

C. Administrative Independence and Separate Budget

1. Administrative independence: If the teaching program is to function as conceived (targeted to education, technical, and investigative experiences), the Program Director must be free to plan for both patient care and learning experiences as interlocking aspects of a holistic approach to each problem-solving endeavor. Independence – freedom – is not licensed, so the bonds between the pediatric Neurosurgery teaching program and the parent Neurosurgery department are by definition firm, with the pediatric aspects being the application of neurosurgical principles to the anatomo-pathological variations which constitute the different ages of childhood (newborn, infant, toddler, juvenile, adolescent). Similarly, pediatric Neurosurgery must be independent of both pediatrics and pediatric surgery.

2. Separate budget: Here, one needs to say no more than that: *without economic independence there is no independence.*

II. Composition

This may be conveniently sub-divided into physical facilities, organizational units, patient load (numbers of patients and operative procedures), and staff.

A. Physical Facilities

These are no different from what we need for any serious, adult – or mixed – neurosurgical unit, nor do the ratios between numbers of operating rooms and numbers of surgical procedures differ. The only differences have to do with equipment specific to the pediatric ages, special accommodations for parents, targeted physical therapy and school facilities.

B. Organizational Units

These are quite distinct, and intricately articulated. The names of the different clinics, which some . . . biting . . . critics could use to chide warmly the pediatric neurosurgeon with the term *subspecialty*, serve the individual disease entities. They also serve the teaching, investigative, and clinical aspects . They are so different one from the other as to require special professional, nursing, psychology, and rehabilitative medicine input. They demand, each of them, totally dedicated social service workers for in-patient and out-patient family assistance. The functional organizational units essential to pediatric Neurosurgery, in order to be able to conceive, conduct, and deliver the education programs which needs must come from a model Fellowship program are:

1. teaching staff,
2. investigative facilities,
3. inpatient services,
4. out patient clinics, and
5. continuing education programs.

1. Teaching staff: as on a general Neurosurgery service, the teachers will invariably range from those who teach by setting an example, performing their art in a human manner and their technical skills consistently with precision, to those who are able to articulate their messages verbally, reducing them to schemata. The teachers cannot be limited to clinical work, for without an investigative arm the teaching program invariably becomes vocational in orientation, taking on the tonality of a trade. This sterilizes the entire educational program, rendering it and its students technicians.

Pediatric Neurosurgery is not a broad enough area of activity to provide a loading dose of clinical and investigative material upon which Fellowship programs may draw to provide regularly new techniques, new information, new perspectives. Consequently, it must bolster these qualitative deficiencies by maintaining constant contact, preferably through direct rotation with a very active, academically oriented, general Neurosurgery program. *Those pediatric Neurosurgery programs which are structurally and functionally isolated within Children's Hospitals cannot and have not generated mature teaching programs capable of functioning along university lines.* This is not meant to imply that excellent, even outstanding, pediatric Neurosurgery may not be performed in these circumstances, but surely that this is not the stuff of a model fellowship program. There is more to it than patients and dedicated clinicians.

2. Investigative facilities: Research, whether it be experimental or clinical, is essential to the formation of all clinical minds, for the physician must learn to evaluate the information available to him, selecting those elements which are solid enough to qualify as evidence, and to organize them consequentially into diagnostic criteria and treatment plans. Above all, he must be able to accept new evidence as it becomes available, tranquilly discarding his previous positions. Given the characteristics and limits of anamneses in children, this assumes major importance in pediatric Neurosurgery. As in all other areas of science, it is not sufficient for staff members to have a research background or to perform investigative studies: there must be research space and an organized program for the Fellows.

3. The in-patient services in pediatric Neurosurgery, apart from the obvious adaptations to the individual age categories, are the same as those for any general neurosurgical program. They should be programmed as direct clinical extension of the Service, dedicated to the care of children, of the parent academic adult department. In fact, they have little in common with other pediatric subspecialties (orthopedics, cardiac surgery, general surgery) and nothing with medical pediatrics, oncology, etc.

4. Outpatient clinics are the very core of pediatric Neurosurgery patient care activities and patient selection. The family still remains the only system, socially and economically capable of providing the full range of support essential to minimize the untoward physical and psychological effects of diseases striking the ages of development. The children need to be treated, rehabilitated, and educated. They must fit into a social system during all phases of their growth ... with their individual disease being faced up to as a reality, from which they may or may not recover completely.

The most important of these clinics are

a. spina bifida
b. epilepsy
c. neuro-oncology
d. hydrocephalus
e. craniofacial anomalies

They are all multidisciplinary clinics, requiring the full participation, at equal levels regarding diagnostic studies and treatment plans, of separate specialists and other health care providers.

5. Continuing education is what separates an academic program that may be ranked among leadership programs, from a training program, which serves the purpose of teaching skills, techniques. Continuing education proceeds along the two lines of ongoing education to the fellows and rotating residents on the one hand, and conducting full-fledged courses for practicing physicians and surgeons, general and pediatric neurosurgeons, health-care professionals and lay volunteers. *Continuing education cannot be left entirely to societies, congresses, Graduate Schools of Education*! I have no intent to be derogatory, for these organizations have a very real role in education, but their role is that of amateurs, those who love what they are doing and do it without pay. Ongoing education in specific subspecialties must also be conducted by the professionals (those who do well what they are paid to do) themselves.

C. Patient Load

In serving a population base of approximately 2,000,000 inhabitants, a pediatric Neurosurgery service will have approximately the following patient load:

1. Outpatients	2,000
2. Inpatients	1,000
3. Surgical procedures	700
– craniotomies	150
– laminotomies	40
– trauma	70
– shunts- insertions	50
revisions	150
– Miscellaneous	150

D. Staff

The just described patient load and the extensively outlined missions for a model pediatric Neurosurgery fellowship will have approximately the following staff:

– Chairman	1
– Associates	2
– Assistants*	2
– Residents	4
– Fellows*	2

It must be stressed that the Residents are those general Neurosurgery residents who rotate through the pediatric Neurosurgery program for a minimum of six [6] months to learn pediatric Neurosurgery, for it is an integral part of Neurosurgery. It is a subspecialty, and should never be considered a free-standing specialty. All neurosurgeons should – must – be familiar enough with pediatric Neurosurgery to be comfortably performing it when the working or geographic conditions make this desirable or necessary. In my opinion, we would make a decisional error to "tack" pediatric Neurosurgery rotations onto the basic clinical program, or to allocate pediatric Neurosurgery post-graduate education to Pediatric Neurosurgery Societies: Neurosurgery is one, its teaching should be one. If there are time constraints, these should be recognized and the programs either lengthened chronologically or condensed conceptually. It is not wise to lop-off entire areas of study such as Pediatrics, Functional, Imaging, Intensive Care. . . . lest we really, and I certainly hope not, consider them true specialties, functionally and structurally different from General Neurosurgery.

Therefore, in this table of organization, I conceive of the Chairman and the two Associates as permanent staff personnel. The two Assistants are, indeed, the pediatric Neurosurgery Fellows, who are taken on as staff personnel and who function in that capacity. They are not to be considered Residents, nor non-descript elements interposed between the Residents and the Staff-Men.

This position immediately begs the most vital questions of all in this essay! "how long should the Fellowship last, and what should the Fellows do?" Since the Fellows are to be brought on for a minimum of two [2] years, and to serve in the capacity of Staff-Men, the duration is variable, depending upon

---

* Assistants are Fellows

personal relationships, service needs, individual career opportunities. Surely, the fellow should already have had a six month rotation through pediatric Neurosurgery during his residency, and he should be a fully qualified neurosurgeon. He should also be of such caliber to be considered eligible for the position of Associate.

Regarding what the fellows should do, the answer is intuitive: pediatric Neurosurgery at a staff level, within the limits of his knowledge, technical skills, and experience.

If, from this essay one concludes that the matter of a Fellowship in Pediatric Neurosurgery is not simple, that it cannot be applied helter-skelter, here and there, that it belongs snugly into a fully accredited and responsibly directed General Neurosurgery academic department, and that it should never become a free-standing specialty, then my presentation will have been a success.

One should also conclude, however, by inductive reasoning, that I think there is no alternative to a Certificate of Special Competence, to be issued by selected academic, University Departments of Neurosurgery or General Neurosurgery Accreditation Boards. A certificate of Special Competence cannot be looked upon to be superior or inferior, in a hierarchical sense, to Residency education and General Neurosurgery board certification.

I suggest that *if we do not make this Certificate available, along lines compatible with our perspectives of Neurosurgery and sub-specialization within, Society and academic anarchists will do so . . . to the detriment of pediatric Neurosurgery, and Neurosurgery.*

III. Conduction

I leave this for the future: a desired time when Neurosurgery will have resolved the problems of sub-specialization, and begun to undertake its implementation.

References

1. Ojemann GA (1993) Subspecialization. American Board of Neurological Surgery Newsletter 13
2. Raimondi AJ (1992) The education and identification of a pediatric neurosurgeon. An essay. Child Nerv Syst 8:4–7
3. Raimondi AJ (1971) The resident and neurosurgery. J Neurosurg [Suppl] 34:286–290
4. Raimondi AJ (1994) Evolution of pediatric neurosurgery as a specialty. Child Nerv Syst 10:353–360
5. Raimondi AJ (1996) The future perspectives of pediatric neurosurgery. Child Nerv Syst 12:59–62
6. Hirsch JF (1995) A department of pediatric neurosurgery in a pediatric hospital. Child Nerv Syst 11:38–40

Correspondence: Prof. A. J. Raimondi, Villa Monteleone, I-37020 Gargagnago (VR), Italy

Acta Neurochir (1997) [Suppl] 69:140–144
© Springer-Verlag 1997

Post Residency Subspecialty Training in Neurosurgery – The Impact of Subspecialty Training on Organized Neurosurgery and Resident Training – Benefits, Responsibilities and Liabilities

D. G. Piepgras

Department of Neurosurgery, The Mayo Clinic, Rochester, Minnesota, U.S.A.

Keywords: Subspecialty training, benefits, liabilities.

Introduction

Currently in the United States there are 113 designated neurosurgical subspecialty fellowships which are directly affiliated with accredited residency training programs (Table 1). Although these fellowships are designated as "available", a number of them are currently inactive. Also, there may exist some "fellowships" which are unaffiliated with residency programs, but there is no reliable information regarding their number or location and such programs are probably insignificant in their potential impact to organized neurosurgery and to resident training.

The designation of "*accredited*" residency programs (of which there are 99 for neurosurgery in the United States) refers to the cyclical process of review and authorization of residency programs by the Accreditation Council for Graduate Medical Education (ACGME) and the specialty specific Residency Review Committee (RRC) to assure that each residency meets the established standards for specialty residency training.

Accredtitation of Fellowships?

The ACGME/residency review process also accredits subspecialty training programs (fellowships) in a multitude of specialties. In neurosurgery, however, the accreditation process has not been extended to cover neurosurgical fellowships, although this would seem logical and appropriate to assure consistency and quality in the subspecialty training experience. There are a number of factors which account for the current non-accreditation of neurosurgical fellowships including:

1) Neurosurgical subspecialty fellowships are relatively new and more time may be necessary before standards for the fellowship training evolve. Such standards must necessarily specify the prerequisite training before entering the fellowship (completion of neurosurgery residency is the usual), the structure of the fellowship, its duration and scope, the spectrum of case material, the faculty requirements and other general educational guidelines.

2) In neurosurgery there are relatively few of each type of fellowship program in part due to neurosurgery being a comparatively small and restricted specialty. In order to justify the accreditation process, it is desirable that there be a "critical mass" of programs. The ACGME has rather arbitrarily specified that there should be a minimum of 25 centers offering training in the subspecialty before an application can be made for accreditation. As already mentioned, in neurosurgery there is only one subspecialty fellowship which is offered at 25 sites, this being in spinal surgery, whereas the others range from one (peripheral nerve) to 19 (neuro-oncology) separate programs. Moreover, many of these designated programs do not maintain a continuously active fellowship, a necessity for accreditation status.

Table 1. *Neurosurgery Subspecialty Fellowships USA 1995–1996*

Cerebrovascular surgery	14
Epilepsy surgery	3
Endovascular surgical neuroradiology	15
Neuro-oncology	19
Neurotrauma & critical care	10
Pediatric neurosurgery	12
Peripheral nerve	1
Spine surgery	25
Skull base surgery	4
Stereotactic & functional neurosurgery	10

3) Finally and probably most important, the American Board of Neurological Surgery (ABNS) and to a large extent practicing neurosurgeons in the U.S. have been opposed to formalization and accreditation of neurosurgery subspecialty training owing to the fear (real or imagined) that a proliferation of accredited subspecialty programs may fragment our relatively small specialty.

Additionally, there is the concern that accredited subspecialty training will ultimately lead to *certification* of those who complete the fellowship training and eventually disenfranchisement of neurosurgeons (even though they may be very well trained in the subspecialty) who do not possess the subspecialty certificate.

The question becomes especially meaningful relative to concerns that subspecialty *certification* could ultimately be used to determine which neurosurgeons may be awarded privileges to perform certain procedures in their hospital or whether a neurosurgeon would be reimbursed for performing a procedure.

Beyond the question of accreditation of fellowships is the issue of whether fellowship training can or should exist without affiliation with an accredited residency program. In the United States there are no rules to this effect and the stipulation would only exist as part of accreditation standards which, as already stated, are not mandatory for fellowship training. In reality, any medical center or group of specialists could develop their own fellowship in a neurosurgical subspecialty and offer it to neurosurgeons without any oversight of curriculum or quality requirements for the faculty.

There are strong arguments for linking subspecialty fellowship training with residency programs, among which are the provision of:

1) An enhanced environment for academic activities.
2) Dedicated faculty including those from other affiliated subspecialties.
3) Opportunities for educational interaction between the fellow and program residents.
4) Existing facilities for clinical or basic research.

Considering these advantages, it is my opinion that if accredited subspecialty training programs were ever to be promulgated in neurosurgery, standards should stipulate for their existence only in conjunction with accredited resident training programs.

Program Benefits of Fellowship Training

Development of a fellowship training program within a department brings certain advantages which include:

1) Augmentation of Clinical Activities

Presumably the fellow will be knowledgeable and experienced (usually a Board eligible neurosurgeon) capable of significantly enhancing the patient care within the department. A well-qualified fellow may function as effectively as a junior staff member who will augment patient care activities on behalf of his neurosurgical mentors and contribute directly to the productivity in the out-patient department, operating room, and postoperative wards.

2) Enhancement of Resident Training and the Academic Program

The fellow should contribute to the resident training and academic program through motivation and mentoring of residents, supervision of residents in patient care both in and out of the operating room. Additionally, the fellow may serve to assist or relieve residents in fulfilling service responsibilities so as to allow the program residents more time for pursuit of academic activities.

3) Recognition of the Department as a Subspecialty Leader

With a successful subspecialty training program, there is likely to be heightened recognition of the department as a leader in the subspecialty owing to its dedicated faculty and research and the associated publications and presentations.

4) Strengthens the Subspecialty

Finally, the subspecialty will be strengthened through the existence of specially trained neurosurgeons dedicated to providing the subspecialty with an enhanced body of knowledge, improved techniques and dedicated research.

Responsibilities and Liabilities

Equally as important to consider in subspecialty training of neurosurgeons are the responsibilities of the directors of this training experience and the realization of the liabilities, the potential risks, which accompany the existence of fellowship training programs.

1) Protection of the Educational Experience of the Program's Residents

Foremost among the liabilities of a fellowship training program is the potential for a negative impact on the overall educational experience of the program's core residents. The inherent danger primarily relates to the potential for competition for operative experience between a fellow and the residents in the program. Programs do exist in the United States where there is open competition between the subspecialty fellow and the program's senior residents for operative experience in select cases. Unless there are adequate cases and the fellowship program is carefully structured and monitored, such competition ultimately results in animosity between the fellow and the program's residents and an adversarial relationship which is directly contrary to an optimal educational environment. In order to minimize the risks for this, the Neurosurgical RRC has recently mandated that before a fellowship can be initiated, it must be demonstrated to the RRC how the fellow will be incorporated into the training program and that there exists adequate case material for training of both resident and fellow. In subsequent reviews of the program, the impact of the fellowship is also examined through review of operative data and confidential and prefererably separate interviews of the program's residents and fellows. Careful attention must be given to assure that the priorities for opera-

tive experience and training go to the residents while still maintaining quality of the fellowship training experience.

2) Provision of a Full Spectrum of Subspecialty Experience

The adequacy of case material must be considered relative to the number of residents in the training program (i.e. one vs. two or even three residents per year) as well as the components that make up the subspecialty training experience (See Figures 1 and 2). For example, in the subspecialty area of pediatric neurosurgery, consideration must be given not simply to the total of pediatric neurosurgery operations

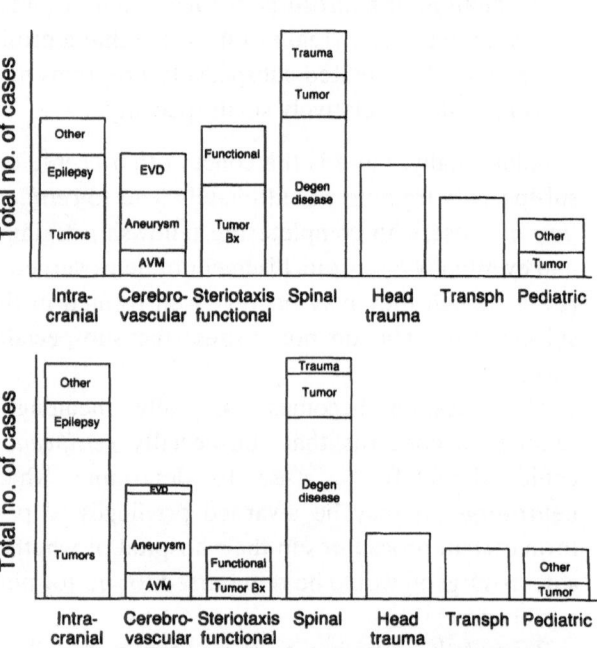

Fig. 1,2. Diagrammatic representation of the spectrum of operative case material for neurosurgery resident training with the annual total number of cases represented on the Y axis and the various categories of operated cases on the X axis. Figure 1 (above) shows a relative balance of cases in the entire spectrum of neurosurgical operations. Depending upon the total number of operations, such a balance could provide adequate training within the program for 1 or 2 residents per year. Figure 2 (down): This graph by comparison shows a less balanced spectrum of operative cases with high numbers of operations for degenerative spine disease and intracranial tumor but relatively few procedures for spinal trauma and extracranial occlusive vascular disease (EVD). The operative case material in this program may be adequate to train 1 resident per year but not 2 given the relative deficiencies in the entire spectrum. Such a program may however adequately provide fellowship training in spinal surgery and/or adult neuro-oncology without adversely impacting the training and operative experience of the program's residents (usually half of which are shunt procedures) but the volume of more complex cases such as pediatric brain tumor, spinal dysraphism and pediatric head injury. Adequate training of either the program's residents or a pediatric neurosurgery fellow in the program cannot be obtained if there is insufficient exposure to all components of the spectrum of pediatric neurosurgery.

A personal example exists in our program at the Mayo Clinic where we have two or three residents at each level of training. In the past, development of focused subspecialty fellowships had been avoided believing that these would interfere with the experience and opportunities of the residents in the program. Recently, and somewhat reluctantly, we joined our Department of Orthopedics in development of a fellowship in spinal surgery. While this fellowship was intended to be a full fellowship in spinal surgery, it has in reality been limited to a fellowship related to the management of degenerative spinal diseases, stabilization and instrumentation, owing to the neurosurgeons' unwillingness to allow participation of the fellow over our own neurosurgical residents in operations for intraspinal neoplasm or other myelopathic conditions. Further, inasmuch as there are a limited number of traumatic spinal injuries at our institution, it has been necessary to develop a protocol which allows participation of the spinal fellow but with the stipulation that he cannot override the participation of the neurosurgery chief resident.

3) Provision of a Structured Curriculum and Dedicated Faculty

Inherent in the offering of the subspecialty training experience is the obligation to provide the trainee a full training experience. The above paragraph gives personal testimony to the difficulties which can be encountered in meeting this laudable obligation to the fellow, who has invested a year of his life for subspecialty training. The subspecialty fellowship should be more than an apprenticeship to a single individual. There must be a well-structured program with a curriculum of conferences and didactic training related to the subspecialty as well as the opportunity for applied research. Additionally, there must be dedicated faculty, preferably not the residency program chairman or resident training director, who will administer the fellowship, mentor

the trainee, and nurture his clinical and professional development.

4) Assure Trainee Quality

For programs establishing and maintaining a subspecialty fellowship, there is an obligation for assuring that the candidates and the selected trainee meet a certain level of excellence. This requirement may prove difficult to meet, but there must be adherence to a quality standard. Subspecialty training should have as its goal the promotion of advanced knowledge and skills necessary for a higher level of excellence and in some cases academic careers for the subspecialist. Fellowships *must not* exist as a remedial school for unqualified or inadequately trained residents. Should there be a limited pool of applicants for fellowship training, there is danger that in order to meet service requirements, an underqualified candidate may be accepted into the fellowship program which may result in a disservice to patients, the sponsoring program, its residents, as well as the subspecialty. If there is a lack of qualified applicants for a fellowship position, it should be the responsibility of both the fellowship director and the program director to leave the position temporarily unfilled or close the fellowship permanently rather than perpetuate proliferation of incapable individuals.

Conclusion

In summary, I would emphasize my opinion that neurosurgery fellowship and subspecialty training carries potential for enhancing the science and art of neurosurgery and the care of our patients. Centers of subspecialty excellence with an abundance of subspecialty case material can foster a high level of focused surgical knowledge, skills, and development of new techniques. Within these centers the fellowship training experience may flourish provided there is a structured curriculum and maintenance of academic standards. Uncontrolled fellowship training without quality standards, a proliferation of fellowship training programs outside of academic institutions or even within residency training programs but without regard to the impact of the fellow, carries potential for harm to neurosurgery and particularly our residents. In neurosurgery, at least for the near future, it also seems desirable that accredited subspecialty training should not be linked to certification of trainees as having special qualifications beyond those of their "generalist" colleagues. Adherence to standards of neurosurgical training should assure that residents are adequately trained in each subspecialty so as to be competent to manage most of the spectrum of neurosurgical diseases.

References

1. Allen WC (1990) The relationship between residency programs and fellowships in the educational setting. Clin Orthop Related Res 257:57–60
2. Anderson KD, Mavis BE (1995) The relationship between career satisfaction and fellowship training in academic surgeons. Am J Surg 169:329–333
3. Crumley RL (1994) Survey of postgraduate fellows in otolaryngology – Head and neck surgery. Arch Otolaryngol Head Neck Surg 120:1074–1079
4. Graduate Medical Education Directory 1996–1997. American Medical Association
5. Miller RH (1994) Otolaryngology residency and fellowship training. The resident's perspective. Arch Otolaryngol Head Neck Surg 120:1057–1061
6. Neurosurgery Subspecialty Fellowships 1995–1996 Directory. Congress of Neurological Surgeons
7. Ojemann RG (1992) Training the neurosurgeon for the twenty-first century. Surg Neurol 37:167–174

Correspondence: D. G. Piepgras, M.D., Department of Neurosurgery, The Mayo Clinic, 200 First Street, SW, 55905 Rochester, Minnesota, U.S.A.

Acta Neurochir (1997) [Suppl] 69:145–150
© Springer-Verlag 1997

In the Realm of Ideas: the Advent of Advanced Surgery of the Human Cerebrum and Neurosurgical Education

M. L. J. Apuzzo

Neurological Surgery and Radiation Oncology, Biology and Physics, University of Southern California School of Medicine, Los Angeles, CA, U.S.A.

Summary

High technology has recently exerted remarkable positive forces within the field of neurological surgery. Striking developments in brain imaging, stereotaxy, molecular biology, radiation physics and complex data management promise to revolutionize surgery of the human cerebrum. These changes are not without profound impact on national health care economics and present enormous philosophical and educational challenges which will create considerable turmoil over the next decades.

Keywords: Health care, computer, cerebral surgery, molecular neurosurgery, stereotaxy, radiosurgery.

I. Introduction

Neurosurgery has enjoyed a remarkable quarter century. Fueled by buoyant economies, popular attitudes and demands and parallel progress in transferable technical and biological areas striking advances have rapidly evolved [5,7,8].

Important trends have included a) a refinement of the preoperative substrate definition, b) miniaturization of operative corridors, c) reduction of operative trauma, d) increased effectiveness at the target site, and e) incorporation of improved technical adjuvants and physical operative tools into treatment protocols.

In particular the computer has become an essential and formidable ally in diagnostic and surgical events.

A concatenation of forces and developments are presenting previously unknown opportunities for surgical enterprises especially within the human cerebrum. These possibilities are heralded by developments related to technical advances in the field.

Four major areas reflect high technology, its current capability and possibility for application [4,8]:

1) *Imaging*, sensors and the concept of visualization as it may be applied to intracranial surgery and relate that to methodology that has come forward from the standpoint of
2) *localization* and *navigation* through the brain
3) *action at the target point* once access has been gained
4) the development of an *operative setting* that might be appropriate to perform whatever operations might be necessary now and in the future.

II. Advanced Imaging Modes

Over the past 25 years there has been a remarkable evolution of the definition of the operative structural substrate with the capabilities of computed tomography, magnetic resonance and ultrasound to provide thousands of data points which may be assembled together in a three-dimensional image formulating either abstractly or on a computer screen a *structural composite* of the operative substrate. Given this composite, one may then develop a "rehearsal" by manipulation of these data points [18].

Recent developments indicate the potential for *functional imaging* that will have the capability of being superimposed on this structural substrate. Echoplanar magnetic resonance is "fast" sequence magnetic resonance or magnetic resonance in a fraction of a second that requires only one nuclear spin excitation per image and maps the blood organ pool, organ profusion, blood flow dynamics and CSF dynamics [1,2]. This methodology not only has the ability to map rudimentary physiological functions but also potentially more complex integrative, associative and cognitive functions.

The concept of superimposition of function on the structural substrate is now emerging into the realm of reality.

Magnetic source imaging represents another sphere of functional imaging. With this method, evoked responses or physiological activity may be measured by flux within magnetic fields through the cranium to define basic functional areas prior to a surgical event. Currently it represents a refined methodology for outlining sensory and motor areas and epileptic foci with more complex methodologies and mapping capabilities promised for the future [13,15].

Optical Imaging represents a fascinating methodology for defining physiological activity. The optical properties of tissues may be measured and enhanced by the utilization of vital dyes and then measuring changes in optical properties as physiological activity takes place. Although it's not certain whether these changes relate to flow of ionic currents, oxygen delivery, blood volume changes, potassium accumulation or glial swelling, the methodology has promise for definition of cortical functional areas. Work in this area has been reported clearly defining the capability of mapping speech areas and epileptigenic foci [16].

These emerging imaging methodologies create a new dimension in a development of preoperative and intraoperative substrates for surgery within the brain and when combined with navigational capabilities, promise to enhance the precision of management of each surgical challenge.

III. Concepts of Navigation

A number of navigational methods have been employed by high technology warfare devices such as submarines. Complex motion sensing gyroscopes may be locked into values of longitude and latitude. They are called "*SINS*" or the Ship's Inertial Navigational Systems. Position may be precisely monitored by movement in a three-dimensional space of water over the surface of the earth. "*LORAIN C*" system is a triangulation methodology for determination of

position by radio wave transmissions. A so-called "*BRN*" system is used to identify satellite reference points which could be superimposed on data from SINS and LORAIN C to further define and reconfirm the accuracy of position. Principles of *celestial navigation* is the most accurate positional reference. Additionally, extensive charts defining the contour of geological formations of the ocean's bottom during a course could be used as reference points, *MODE G*.

Therefore, a combination of navigational based methodologies are employed to ensure absolute determination of a ship's position at all times, and it is apparent that a number of similar methodologies have been employed in the field of stereotactic neurosurgery to determine anatomical position based on three dimensional imaging maps [8].

IV. Cerebral Stereotaxy

Twenty years ago work began with single planes in stereotactic space relating single points to external fiducials to do what was in fact a "point" stereotactic surgery. With more complex computer application, we progressed into a concept of "volume" stereotaxis. A new era opened by taking thousands of imaging data points, placing them in stereotactic space in volumetric systems, changing view lines to opportunistic settings and then using imaging-guided stereotaxy in a volumetric system to deal through safe functional corridors to deep brain lesions [20,22].

The concept of "non-linkage" was initiated by the Dartmouth/Hanover Group where an amalgam was established between scalp *fiducials* for localization through imaging, a series of *spark gaps* that were placed on a microscope stand and *microphones* in the ceiling of an operating room so that the room, per se, became the stereotactic instrument [24]. A union was established between intracranial space and representative images whereby the microscope could then be localized in planes of action with a secondary cathode ray tube on the side of the microscope being employed as a visual guide to navigate through the patient's brain with absolute recognition to the focal points of plane.

These concepts were carried forward with the development of three-dimensional digitalizers in the seminal work by Watanabe and Takakura at the University of Tokyo – work which has given impetus to a number of different concepts related to digit-alizers [12,27].

Currently various systems employ jointed digitalizers, light emitting diodes, magnetic field digitalizers, inertial navigation and radio frequency time delay systems that can be locked into stereotactic space either by fiducials placed on the scalp, skull or utilization of laser scanners to define the geometric pattern of the skull and then register it in stereotactic space so that a complexly instrumented microscope can be used to navigate through the brain and perineural areas [8].

V. A Spectrum of Target Point Action

Following refinement of navigational maps and transitional capability, the question arises "What happens at the target point?"

The principal action at the target point continues to be removal of tissue. There is no doubt that microdissection methods will continue to be central. In many cases, dependent on the progress of endovascular techniques, application of an aneurysm clip and other events will continue.

However, new dimensions of ablation through use of radiant energy and capabilities for functional restoration provide us with exciting vistas and areas to be explored.

1) Ablation

The concept of *stereotactic radiosurgery* is central. Its methods and capabilities may be considered under the title of application of "high energy forms" in neurological surgery [8,21].

Heavy particles have been used for a period of time taking advantage of the Bragg Peak and attenuation of energy waves by certain modifiers. There is variability according to types of particles that are used associated with variables of effective oxygenation, dose distribution and linear energy transfer. The employment of these heavy particles requires massive instruments with installation costs as high as 40 million dollars, thus the practicality of utilization is not high.

A significant breakthrough emerged with the genesis of the concept of employing *rotational* capabilities of gantry and couch incorporated in hospital-based *linear accelerator* systems and coupling this with point stereotaxy isolating the target

point with a volume-type setting and then producing a photon influx creating a volumetric isolated energy transfer.

Certainly, one of the most important creative concepts was developed by Lars Lexell in the '50s with the fixed-beam cobalt-60 sources aligned in an arc centered system. The current generation of gamma unit devices represents an elegant amalgam of physics, mechanics and computer science. At this time 25 *Gamma Units* are in operation in the United States, and approximately 70 worldwide.

The concept of the *free electron laser* may offer a new and valuable dimension. This laser methodology was predicated on the physical concept of generation of laser energy by an electron being accelerated through a series of magnetic fields. These magnetic fields can be varied and depending on the amount of energy applied, variation in the wave length of monochromatic light is realized. One then has the ability of having virtually a large portion of the electromagnetic spectrum available for clinical application. This system allows for not only multiple frequencies but also ultra-short pulses and ultra-high intensities capable by this principle – all desirable qualities for an optimum laser instrument for neurological surgery.

The *photodynamic therapies* (PDT) which have had some difficulties in practical application may be enhanced by the introduction of this free-electron laser type of instrumentation in an operating room setting. Photoreactive dyes are given intravenously. They tend to establish a capture net in neoplasms, infected and embryological tissues. Monochromatic red light effects a coagulation necrosis. There are problems with dye accumulations and the uniformity of capture nets, therefore more effective types are needed. Additionally, problems exist with penetration of red light which acts as the photoreactive catalyst. With improvements in capabilities of biochemistry and physical applications such as the free electron laser, it is feasible to envision a type of combined methodology where stereotactic principles may be applied in conjunction with a free electron laser and photodynamic dyes for the management of neoplastic and focal infectious disorders [8].

There has been a renaissance of interest in *BORON Capture Therapy* [14]. The element boron serves as a capture net for thermal (slow) neutrons. About 70 patients were treated during the decade of the '50s, but technical improvements are required. There has been further research initiated by the development of a more satisfactory boron compound in Japan, and now there is *boron phenylalanine* which coupled with a more energetic thermal neutron source at the Brookhaven National Laboratory is felt to offer promise as an investigational methodology for management of intrinsic gliomas.

VI. Cellular/Molecular Neurosurgery and Functional Restoration

There is no doubt that the concept of *functional restoration* in the nervous system, and especially as embodied in the term "molecular or cellular neurosurgery" offers an exciting window and far reaching possibility for the future [8,28,29]. We were active from the standpoint of adrenal medullary autografts and were encouraged by the results of our series [3]. A central problem in the field was the capability of maintaining viability of cells that were grafted. Currently, it is clear that very major improvements are imminent. In *Science* a review has recently described three articles that had occurred in *Nature, Cell* and *Nature Medicine* [11]. These described methodologies that demonstrated that co-culture of embryonic cells from a midbrain with fibroblasts that had been genetically engineered to secrete a fibroblast growth factor would significantly enhance graft viability over an extended period of time.

In addition, other data showed the ability to use primitive floorplate cells in culture with undifferentiated neural precursor cells to induce an evolution of dopaminergic neurons negating the requirement for large numbers of fetuses as donors.

And, finally, and perhaps most exciting, there was noted a report from Genetec Laboratories that one could use the principle of using genetically engineered glial-derived growth factor directly into a region to restore function.

A variety of genetically engineered fragments hold hope for functional restoration, treatment of brain tumors or management of stroke [28,29].

These promising innovative methodologies may be employed with stereotactic methods or techniques that alter the blood brain barrier.

VII. Developments in the Operative Venue

In consideration of these imaginative trends, it would seem that attention to *operating room* design is in order. Therefore, some years ago we embarked on a plan to establish a dedicated, self-contained computerized operating room setting that gave the capability for micro-operative and stereo-operative surgery that was both integrated and complex. We established an amalgam that was both practical and a "think tank" among the Jet Propulsion Laboratory (JPL), the School of Cinema Television, the School of Medicine and the School of Engineering all at the University of Southern California. A complex *Windows on the Human Brain* project was directed to augment, design and develop an operating room setting that would be avant-garde setting the stage as an operating laboratory, taking advantage of many of the principles and concepts that were evolving in a futuristic pattern.

The culmination of these efforts was an operative venue highlighted by a computer-based visualization system that was documented in *Neurosurgery* [6] the heart of the platform was a three-station visualization laboratory for image processing, graphics management and rehearsal of surgeries [8]. This system has provided the capability to very practically perform neurosurgeries from a micro and stereotactic point of view while recording and enhancing their teaching elements.

As such concepts evolve, there is no question that we will be moving into an area of the practical employment of *virtual reality* in the operating room or a setting for rehearsal and training [25]. This is a method to visualize, manipulate and interact with a computer system in which ultimately one has an envelope of immersion in a three-dimensional world. Sensors for movement tracking, computers and optical systems are used to create this illusionary system. There are currently volumes of literature and energetic research activity in this area. This work indicates that virtual reality and the introduction of virtual reality into the operating room and operating room training and rehearsal is currently happening in many other fields and is destined to influence neurosurgery. In addition, there can be integration between the concept of operating room virtual reality and *robotic systems*.

It is apparent that in stereotactic methods concepts are being developed that include voice control in the operating room, real time holograms and robotics. Robotics can reduce operative trauma through reduction of surgical tremor. The best surgeon presumably has a tremor of about 40 microns. With robotic systems, that can be reduced to 4 microns. In theory, virtual reality can be used in combination with robotic systems for more precise surgery.

In consideration of creative developments and advances, the impetus for diverse progress relates to integration of technical aspects from various fields. It has been the combination and cross fertilization from seemingly unrelated and "remote areas" that has made the unusual and innovative a reality.

VIII. Educational Considerations

These striking developments are attended by profound philosophical and economic considerations [8,10,17,26].

The cost of effecting such advances is enormous. Globally national economies are restricted with demands for limits on components of gross national products devoted to health care. These developments and requirements have and are impacting upon elements of research, development and training.

Questions of who will be trained in advanced methods, how they will be trained, how will competence be measured and who will be treated are thorny problems that have no easy answers.

Software development is particularly costly and has slowed ambitious plans as economic constraints make their presence felt.

A bright spot would appear to be the relatively economical availability of the INTERNET and WORLDWIDE WEB as a communications network and methodology [19,23]. This reality for rapid economic and advanced communication is already affecting neurosurgery and all medical disciplines by accelerating information transfer in rapid order as a splendid development of the computer age. It has only been minimally explored as a vehicle for education but will no doubt be essential to all in the future.

References

1. Alper J (1993) Innovation in imaging Echo Planar MRI: learning to read minds. Science 261:556
2. Alper J (1933) Innovation in imaging EEG + MRI: a sum greater than the parts. Science 261:559
3. Apuzzo MLJ, Neal JH, Waters CH, Appley AJ, Boyd SD, Couldwell WT, Wheelock VH, Weiner LP (1990) Utilization of unilateral and bilateral stereotactically placed adrenomedullary-striatal autografts in parkinsonian humans: rationale, techniques and observations. Neurosurgery 26,5:746–757
4. Apuzzo MLJ, Chin LS, Chen T, Valencia P (1992) Neurosurgery: a futuristic prospectus. Neurosurgery for the third millennium. Neurosurgical topics. American Association of Neurological Surgeons, Parkridge, IL, pp 11–23
5. Apuzzo MLJ (1992) (ed) Neurosurgery for the third millennium. Neurosurgical topics. American Association of Neurological Surgeons, Parkridge, IL
6. Apuzzo MLJ, Weinberg RA (1993) Architecture and functional design of advanced neurosurgical operating environments. Neurosurgery 33,4:663–673
7. Apuzzo MLJ (1995) Evolving dimensons at the frontiers of human cerebral surgery. Benign cerebral glioma, vol II. Neurosurgical topics. American Association of Neurological Surgeons, Parkridge, IL, pp 1–12
8. Apuzzo MLJ (1996) The Richard C. Schneider Lecture New dimensions of neurosurgery in the realm of high technology: possibilities, practicalities, realities. Neurosurgery 38,4:625–639
9. Aukstakalnis S, Blatner D (1992) SILICON MIRAGE. The art and science of virtual reality. Peachpit Press, Berkeley, CA
10. Awad IA (1995) Philosophy of neurological surgery. Neurosurgical topics. American Association of Neurological Surgeons, Park Ridge, IL
11. Barinaga M (1995) Researchers broaden the attack on Parkinson's disease. Science 267:455–456
12. Barnett GH, Kormos DW, Steiner CP, Weisenberg J (1993) Use of a frameless, armless stereotactic wand for brain tumor localization with two-dimensional and three-dimensional neuroimaging. Neurosurgery 33,4:674–678
13. Benzel EC, Lewine JD, Bucholz RD, Orrison WW Jr (1993) Magnetic source imaging: a review of the Magnes system of Biomagnetic Technologies Incorporated. Neurosurgery 33,2:252–259
14. Flam F (1994) Will history repeat for boron capture therapy? Science 265:468–469
15. Gallen CC, Sobel DF, Waltz T, Aung M, Copeland B, Schwartz BJ, Hirschkoff EC, Bloom FE (1993) Noninvasive presurgical neuromagnetic mapping of somatosensory cortex. Neurosurgery 33,2:260–268
16. Haglund MM, Ojemann GA, Hochman DW (1992) Optical imaging of epileptiform and functional activity in human cerebral cortex. Nature 358:668–671
17. Hegel GWF (1917–1920) Vorlesungen über die Philosophie der Weltgeschichte. Felix Meiner, Leipzig
18. Hu X, Tan KK, Levin DN, Galhotra S, Mullan JF, Hekmatpanah J, Spire J-P (1990) Three-dimensional magnetic resonance images of the brain: application to neurosurgical planning. J Neurosurg 72:433–440
19. Kim R, Kelly PJ (1996) Applications of the World Wide Web to neurosurgical practice. Neurosurgery 39,6:1169–1182
20. Koivukangas J, Louhisalmi Y, Alakuijala, Oikarinen J (1993) Ultrasound-controlled neuronavigator-guided brain surgery. J Neurosurg 79:36–42
21. Luxton G, Petrovich Z, Jozsef G, Nedzi LA, Apuzzo MLJ (1993) Stereotactic radiosurgery: principles and comparison of treatment methods. Neurosurgery 32,2:241–259
22. Morita A, Kelly PJ (1993) Resection of intraventricular tumors via a computer-assisted volumetric stereotactic approach. Neurosurgery 32,6:920–927
23. Pareras LG, Martin-Rodriguez JG (1996) Neurosurgery and the Internet: a critical analysis and a review of available resources. Neurosurgery 39,1:216–233
24. Roberts DW, Strohbehn JW, Hatch JF, Murray W, Kettenberger H (1986) A frameless stereotaxic integration of

computerized tomographic imaging and the operating microscope. J Neurosurg 65:545–549

25. Satava RM, Morgan K, Sieburg HB, Mattheus R, Christensen
JP (1995) Interactive technology and the new paradigm for
healthcare. IOS Press, Washington DC

26. Van Der Meulen JP (1994) Can academic health centers survive health care reform? Neurosurgery 35,4:725–731

27. Watanabe E, Mayanagi Y, Kosugi Y, Manaka S, Takakura K
(1991) Open surgery assisted by the neuronavigator, a stereotactic, articulated, sensitive arm. Neurosurgery 28,6:792–800

28. Zlokovic BV, Apuzzo MLJ (1996) Cellular and molecular
neurosurgery: pathways from concept to reality, part I. Targets and concept approaches in gene therapy of the central
nervous system. Neurosurgery (in press)

29. Zlokovic BV, Apuzzo MLJ (1996) Cellular and molecular
neurosurgery: pathways from concept to reality, part II. Vec-
tor systems and delivery methodologies for gene therapy of
the central nervous system. Neurosurgery (in press)

Correspondence: M. L. J. Apuzzo, M.D., Neurological Surgery
and Radiation Oncology, Biology and Physics, University of
Southern California School of Medicine, 1200 North State Street,
Room 5046, Los Angeles, California 90033, U.S.A.

Acta Neurochir (1997) [Suppl] 69:151–155
© Springer-Verlag 1997

The Development of Training Systems in General Surgery

G. Buess

Chirurgische Klinik, Klinikum Schnarrenberg, Universität Tübingen, Federal Republic of Germany

Keywords: Training systems in surgery, plastic trainers with integrated organs, virtual-reality trainer.

1. Introduction

Endoscopic Surgery was introduced in general surgery particularly during the last 10 years. In the early eighties, only a small number of specialists used endoscopes to perform surgical tasks, whereas in 1996 endoscopic operative procedures, as for instance cholecystectomy, became standard therapy. The training of the endoscopic surgeon therefore became a major task to guarantee safe introduction of the new operative technique into clinical routine.

The hands-on courses in the United States have mainly been performed by working with animals. Although the anatomy of the pig differs considerably from the anatomic situation in humans, this animal was chosen for standard training due to practical aspects and psychological conditions preventing, for example, the work with dogs.

The advantages of the animal model are that ventilation and perfusion are present during the operation so that all techniques of hemostasis can be trained. The disadvantage of this method is that it is expensive, that the anatomical conditions are different, and that therefore the time for practical training is very much restricted and the amount of practical training reduced to a few hours a day.

The disadvantags of the animal model were the reason that our group focused from the very beginning on simulation for training. In 1985 we started courses for training Transanal Endoscopic Microsurgery (TEM). Performing these courses, plastic trainers were equipped with animal organs. This technique of simulation by the use of animal organs from the slaughterhouse has been more and more established during the last 10 years.

The future technique of simulation will become more abstract. Interactive treatment of three-dimensional virtual images by the use of specific training phantoms allows simulating human anatomy, elasticity and bleeding without using real organs. This technique is used today already for flight simulation and will be integrated in the education of the surgeon within the next years.

2. History of Courses

The basis of today's course system applied in Tübingen was developed after clinical introduction of the different endoscopic techniques. The author of this article had at that time very limited pre-experience from different courses in micro-surgery and arthroscopy which took place before 1980.

The first MIC technique introduced in general surgery was named transanal endoscopic microsurgery (TEM), and was developed by our group at the Department of General Surgery at the University of Cologne. After clinical introduction of this procedure, it soon became apparent that surgeons who wanted to adopt this rather difficult technique had no chance to start this activity in a safe way by following the above-mentioned conventional rules of skills education. Therefore we started with the development of the first course system for TEM in 1984 [1].

Those courses for TEM that started in 1985 had been developed independently of the work of Semm in Kiel [2]. The first courses were organised as most of the courses during the 1980s: the equipment was built up at the clinic and the course performed by the personnel from the clinic, i.e. the doctors and medical technical assistants involved in the development work. Close cooperation was maintained with the people from industry, for instance Manfred Böbel, who had been doing most of the development work for the TEM technique [3,4].

Following discussions with the university we decided in 1990 to start a professional training center as a non-profit institution. The concept was that instrumentation and other equipment was sponsored by industry, and the running costs of the courses (payment of the tutors and course material) had to be financed by the fees of the course participants. Starting sponsors from industry were Wolf (Knittlingen), Ethicon (Norderstedt) and AutoSuture (Tönisvorst).

Considering the TEM courses, the number of participants from German speaking countries is decreasing because a significant number of surgeons is already educated in this technique. On the other side we see a rise in participants from foreign countries, a sign that TEM today has an increasing application internationally. TEM courses today are also being held in Great Britain, the USA, and Japan.

At the moment we experience the establishment of task and technology orientated courses. This means that routine operative tasks as cholecystectomy or fundoplication are performed in an experimental setting, and new technology like operative room systems or camera guiding systems is used by the course members.

3. The Different Educational Tools

Today, a wide variety of different tools are available for training of manual skills and of more or less complete operative procedures. In different countries different concepts were preferred in the past whereas today there seems to be a tendency towards generally accepted procedures.

3.1 Animal Experiments

From the very beginning the animal experiment was the dominating educational tool in the United States [5]. The advantage of this concept is that no specific preparation is necessary and no long-lasting development work must be performed before starting courses. Other advantages are that aspects like placing the trokars, dissecting blood vessels, movement of the organs in dependance of the ventilation are comparable to a real clinical operation [6].

On the other side there are definite disadvantages of animal experiments:

- relatively expensive
- extensive preparation
- anesthesia necessary
- more or less anatomical differences to the human situation
- limited time available for the different steps of the operation, which makes didactic teaching more difficult

3.2 Plastic Trainers

During the last years, intensive development work has been performed by structuring body forms with realistic human anatomical design and specific plastic organs, coming close to the anatomical conditions concerning colour and consistency. The leading company in this area is *Limbs and Things* from Bristol, which has done extensive development work resulting in the construction of "close-to-reality" models of human anatomy.

The disadvantages of this model are as follows:

- Dissection in most situations does not come close to reality
- Frequent application in a realistic way is not possible
- Simulation of bleeding is not possible
- High costs of disposable organs

3.3 Plastic Trainers with Integrated Animal Organs

This model is a compromise between the above-mentioned concepts. It has the advantage that relations between spaces and the neighbouring structures are close to reality of human anatomy. Also, the quality of simulation with animal organs (from the slaughterhouse) is much closer to reality than with plastic models. Another advantage is that expenses with this system are relatively low so that surgical tasks can be repeated as often as necessary, which is important when training skills in beginners (Fig. 1).

The disadvantages of this system are as follows:

- Simulation of bleeding not possible.

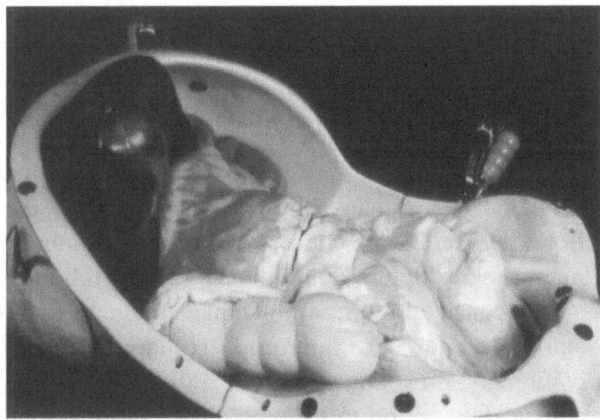

Fig. 1. Liver form with integrated pig's liver, gall bladder and duct system from the slaughterhouse

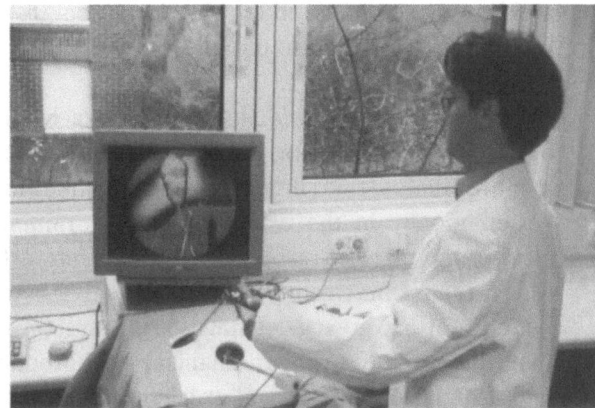

Fig. 2. Karlsruhe simulator for laparoscopic cholecystectomy

3.4 Plastics Trainers with Integrated Perfused Animal Organs

When harvesting the organs from the slaughterhouse under specific circumstances, a perfusion of the organs with differently coloured solutions is possible by using roller pumps [7]. Optimal conditions were found for the perfusion of animal colon. Large vessels show a quite natural bleeding situation and ligations can be performed in a realistic way. We have not been successful in achieving an acceptable perfusion of the bowel wall and the mucosal layer itself. This concept would have been an important aspect for TEM simulation.

The disadvantages are:

– Extensive preparation work of the model
– Not possible for all organs

3.5 Computer Simulation

Development performed together with Kühnapfel from the research center in Karlsruhe [8] is based on the use of high-speed computers (Silicon Graphics – Onyx) in combination with a software generated in the research center (KISMET), and the use of a specifically constructed trainer. This trainer is equipped with instrument handles and a camera body (Fig. 2). The movements of the instruments are measured by an integrated technique which are then transformed into the three-dimensional anatomy using simulated instrument movements. This simulation is a true virtual reality condition; this means that real interactive work inside the computer simulated three-dimensional structures is possible. Meanwhile we

could reach a close-to-reality dissection of the gallbladder, clipping of the cystic duct and a transsection using scissors. Instrument changes can easily be performed by programming the instrument via a foot pedal. Similar developments are going on in the USA [9,10].

Disadvantages of the computer simulation:

– Equipment extremely expensive at present
– Only limited modelling of three-dimensional anatomy available for performing surgical tasks

3.6 Discussion

Procedure related training is a relatively new approach for education in surgery. Specific hands-on courses have been developed in order to adopt various endoscopic procedures. The training systems have improved and are the result of flexible reactions to practical needs. This article describes briefly the situation existing today and some planned solutions for the future.

3.6.1 Structures for Training

In most institutions involved in the training of surgeons, no structures have been existing for the specific training necessary when starting with endoscopic surgery. For practical and economic reasons the establishment of training centers is recommended where surgeons from a larger area can come together for education and specific courses. The need for concentration of training together with the fact that in Germany from the side of the medical societies or state organisations no structures and no personnel have been dedicated to this educational task, resulted in the following solutions:

1. *Company-based educational centers:* As a result of the rising market for instruments and equipment for endoscopic surgery, some companies invested money in the establishment of training centers, thereby also respecting their own interest, to use the training centers as very effective marketing tools. A great advantage of this system is that due to the stronger financial background high-standard buildings and excellent equipment allow very convenient and effective training. Specific personnel that is professionally focusing upon the educational tasks guarantees an optimal organisation and professional advice. The disadvantage of the company-based structure is the specific product orientation which means that only products from the own company or allied companies are used. This results in a strong bias, for example, towards disposable instruments used by most of the education centers. It is therefore often not possible to use effective, probably better products produced by competing companies.

2. *Clinic-based education:* Courses organized by clinical institutions, without long-term commitment to training have been the main educational tool during the introduction of new procedures. The advantage of this structure is that it can react highly flexibly on actual needs, and specifically allows that personal experience of a surgeon with a new technique can immediately and personally be taught. The disadvantages of such structures are that an optimal organisation and precise didactic principles mostly cannot be guaranteed because of the lack of educational routine and the lack of trained education personnel.

3. *Dedicated training centers:* In our opinion, it would be best to build up an educational structure including professional personnel for educational tasks at a neutral place, such as a university or another clinical structure. This structure would also need the financial support of companies involved in the production of different equipment. However, an independent training center can maintain a neutral position and allow new upcoming products from competing companies to be integrated into the courses. Another great advantage would be that close interaction between training in the center and a clinical hospitation may be organised.

3.6.2 Who Should be Trained?

The question whether training courses are necessary to prepare surgeons for the performance of endoscopic operations, which are routinely done in the clinical institutions, presently is debated controversially. In Germany, there is a tendency to continue the traditional concept of no prior training of manual skills before doing the clinical operation.

We consider it preferable that surgeons before starting a new procedure like fundoplication or colorectal procedures should attend a training course. The option to train manual skills at optimal didactic conditions and supervision in a quiet and concentrated surrounding can positively be usd [11]. During the training course the operative tasks can be repeated as often as necessary. In our basic course, for example, one group of three surgeons performs 18 to 24 cholecystectomies and we can recognize a clear learning curve concerning speed of operation and reduction of gall bladder perforations with each day of training.

3.6.3 Which Training Concept Should be Used?

During the last years, a variety of training modalities have been established. For each specific course the optimal training model should be selected; this means different training concepts are matching different situations.

A critical discussion in this context must be focused on the use of animals. The above presented principle of combining artificial human anatomy with animal organs (with or without perfusion) is matching most tasks, particularly in gastrointestinal surgery, better than the animal. The human anatomy is supplied by the training model and the animal organs are well integrated into the anatomical training situation [12]. We are convinced that operations on living animals should only be performed when other training concepts do not render optimal conditions for reaching the goal of training. Operations on animals should therefore be restricted to operations where the conditions of the beating heart are necessary, i.e. training of cardiac bypass or surgical reconstruction of larger vessels.

3.6.4 Future Perspectives

For the education of pilots most of the training is performed in a "virtual reality trainer" i.e. a flight simulator. A similar development may be anticipated for the education in surgery. Based on training systems, as developed together with the research center in Karlsruhe, three-dimensional anatomic models will have to be structured for all anatomical areas. Interactive trainers may then be used to perform the different surgical procedures in a simulated or virtual environment. The prerequisites to establish such training are present today. The dataset for three-dimensional anatomy as well as work stations (for example Silicon Graphics, Onyx) – though expensive – are available and the virtual training box is ready for use.

Above all it is a political task to convince the people providing grants for research and education that this concept of training will be very important in many disciplines. We anticipate that a simple model of a trainer box will be used by medical students to learn human anatomy in a very logical and effective way, i.e. by guiding the camera through the abdomen, and by using a simple rod for palpation so that organs can be moved and the optic can look behind the different structures. As a next step, human pathology can be taught by this tool and finally all conventional surgical procedures as well as endoscopic or radiologic interactive procedures can be simulated in a perfect way. Furthermore, operations may be simulated respecting specific patients' data. As an example, the CT-scan of a patient with rectal cancer could be integrated in the trainer dataset and the surgeon could perform the critical steps of this operation the day before in a realistic simulation so that he would be optimally prepared for the operation itself.

3.6.5 Perspectives for the Use of Simulation in Neurosurgery

In contrast to general surgery, where the actual position of anatomical areas is highly dependent on the state of ventilation and the positioning of the patient, neurosurgical anatomy is embedded in bony structures ensuring a higher stability of the position. This allows to define precisely the anatomy of a lesion as well as important surrounding anatomic structures by using modern imaging techniques like CT or MRI.

Consequently, neurosurgery offers optimal preconditions for the simulation of surgical interventions.

Two levels of simulation might be established:

1. *Standard pathologies:* CT- or MR-scans of frequent tumor locations can be used to be transformed into a three-dimensional construction. Operation of these tumors can be simulated by the use of a computer-linked training phantom.
2. *Training of individual operations:* Computer programmes can be developed to allow the individual anatomy of a lesion being integrated into the three-dimensional computer model. Thus the surgeon can train and analyse the optimal sequence of steps for the individual operation the day before the operation. In conclusion, training of surgical interventions will, in the near future, be increasingly performed by the use of computer simulation. The particular situation in neurosurgery is favourable for this purpose.

References

1. Kipfmüller K, Mentges B, Lattwein G, Hack D, Bueß G (1990) Das videogestützte Kurssystem zur transanalen endoskopischen Mikrochirurgie In: Bueß G (Hrsg) Endoskopie. Deutscher Ärzte-Verlag, Köln, S 344–347
2. Semm K (1990) Ausbildung für die endoskopische Mikrochirurgie. In: Bueß G (Hrsg) Endoskopie. Deutscher Ärzte-Verlag, Köln, S 339 ff
3. Kipfmüller K, Bueß G, Naruhn M, Junginger T (1988) Training program for transanal endoscopic microsurgery. Surg Endoscop 2:24–27
4. Bueß G, Cuschieri (1994) Training in endoscopic surgery. In: Cuschieri A, Bueß G, Périssat J (eds) Operative manual of endoscopic surgery. Springer, Berlin Heidelberg New York Tokyo, pp 64–83
5. Böhm B, Milsom JW (1994) Animal models as educational tools in laparoscopic colorectal surgery. Surg Endoscop 8:707–713
6. Szabo Z, Biggerstaff ED, Kelly NJ, Woy W. Designing an advanced laparoscopic surgery training center. Surgical Technology International IV
7. Szinicz G, Beller S, Bodner W, Zerz A, Glaster K (1993) Simulated operations by pulsatile organ-perfusion in minimally invasive surgery. Surg Laparoscop Endoscop 3, 4:315–317
8. Kühnapfel UG, Neisius B (1993) CAD-Based graphical computer simulation in endoscopic surgery. End Surg 1:181–184

Correspondence: Prof. Dr. G. F. Buess, Abteilung Allgemeine Chirurgie und Poliklinik, Chirurgische Klinik, Klinikum Schnarrenberg, Universität Tübingen, Koppe-Seyler-Strasse 3, D-72076 Tübingen, Federal Republic of Germany

Acta Neurochir (1997) [Suppl] 69:156–157

Interactive Multimedia Software for Training and Education in Neurosurgery

M. M. Batschkus

IBE – Institut für Medizinische Informationsverarbeitung, Biometrie und Epidemiologie, München, Federal Republic of Germany

Summary

Medicine with its abundance of facts and richness of imaging techniques has always been adopting new technologies to improve teaching and training. As a natural consequence, the use of computer-based multimedia technology is generally increasing in medicine and also reaching the field of neurosurgery. Especially the use of interactive multimedia technology seems promising to improve training and education and increase accessibility of highly specific material.

Keywords: Interative multimedia, interactive training, simulation of situations, electronic atlas, organ based programs.

Software Categories and Examples

The software that can be used in neurosurgical training and teaching can be divided into several categories. This is by no means a complete compilation but rather a survey of the most frequent and useful major categories. All mentioned programs have been installed and proved their usefulness in our Multimedia Learning Center at Großhadern University Hospital.

Electronic Atlases

This category transfers traditional atlases into electronic media offering to the user and publisher several advantages: First, they are often easier to navigate and images are accessible by keywords. Second, only the needed information (e.g. the name of a specific structure) is displayed, thus minimizing possible confusion. Third, and this is true for all electronic publications, they are easier to update and cheaper to publish and distribute. Additionally, some new technologies allow 3D orientation and -manipulation of objects.

Examples for this category are "Neurological Atlas", "The Digital Anatomist – Interactive Brain Atlas" and "3-D Brain".

Reference Materials/Electronic Books

These programs do not overflow with typical multimedia material like images, movies and sound. Their strength is to make a large body of text (with or without image) easily and uniquely accessible through hyperlinks and powerful search engines.

Examples for this category, though not specific for neurosurgery are the "Stedman's Medical Dictionary" and the "Merck Manual".

Simulations

With increasing speed of desktop computers even this former by exclusive software category becomes available and affordable. Depending on the used program different methods, conditions or procedures can be experienced more or less like in real life. Traditionally, medical learning takes place predominantly in real situations. Unfortunately not all desirable situations can be offered for training and education (e.g. special patients). Simulations try to fill this gap. Furthermore learning can adopt a playful attitude and scenarios can be trained in a systematic way or as a self test with a random component. Examples for this type of programs are "Advanced Cardiac Life Support", "Lazy Eye" and "Surgeon III – The Brain".

Organ System Based Programs

There are only a few programs trying to accomodate all aspects of a complete organ system under one interface. Relevant to neurology and neurosurgery is "HyperBrain" produced by the University of Utah. The scope ranges from very basic neuroanatomy and neurophysiology to more advanced neuropathology and clinical aspects. Due to its connection to the "Slice of Brain" videodisk and the already mentioned "Interactive Brain Atlas", the richness of image material and information of "HyperBrain" is overwhelming.

Conclusion

For several reasons it might be particularly useful to integrate computer-based multimedia programs into teaching and training in neurosurgery Visualization and free manipulation of three-dimensional representations of neuroanatomical structures make it easier to grasp complex contexts. Teachers and trainers therefore gain time for essential advanced educational tasks that the computer cannot perform. Image rich reference material can easily and more economically be offered in a standardized way than traditional print media or video. Recent advances in network technology allow distribution over the departmental or hospital network. In the lecture hall multimedia technology and software allows flexible use of text, images, animations and digital movies and enables the lecturer to vary his presentation and to address questions or momentary needs.

Addresses

"Advanced Cardiac Life Support", "Critical Care Simulator" and others.
Anesoft Corp.
Issaquah, WA
Fax (206) 643-0092

"Brain 3D".
Martin Rydmark

University Göteborg, Sweden
Fax ++46-31-7733758

"The Digital Anatomist – Interactive Brain Atlas".
University of Wahington
Health Sciences Center for Educational Resources
T-252, Health Sciences Building, SB-56
Seattle, Washington 98195
http://www1.biostr.washington.edu/da/DAProgram.html
Email: bolles@u.washington.edu

"HyperBrain", "Lazy Eye" and an extensive selection of other medical software.
University of Utah
Eccles Health Sciences Library Bldg.589
Salt Lake City, UT 84112
Fax: (801) 582-2623
Email: amthelin@medlib.med.utah.edu

"Merck Manual" and an extensive selection of other medical software.
Keyboard Publishing
482 Norriston Road
Bluebell, PA 19422
Fax: (610) 832-0948
http://www.kbpub.com/default.htm

"Multimedia Learning Center" (Multimedia-Lerncenter-Medizin) at Großhadern University Hospital.
URL: http://www.med.uni-muenchen.de/ibe/mmlc/mmlc.html

"Surgeon III – The Brain".
ISM, Inc.
2103 Harmony Woods Road
Owing Mills, MD 21117
Fax: (410) 560-1306

Correspondence: Dr. med. M. M. Batschkus, IBE – Institut für Medizinische Informationsverarbeitung, Biometrie und Epidemiologie, Marchioninistrasse 15, D-81377 München, Federal Republic of Germany

Index of Keywords

Accreditation 83
Annual acceptance 40
Austria 73
Automotive industry 19

Benefits 140
Breach of standard 101
British Isles 36

Calculation model 40
Categories of research 106
Cerebral surgery 145
Certification 83
Clinical research 116
Clinical trials 116
Competency training 58
Computer 145
Contents 70
Criteria 22

Denmark 40

Education 40
Electronic atlas 156
Energy 12
European examination 89
Evaluation of teaching 98
Examination 93
Examinations training program 98
Experience 89

Failure of residency training 101

Germany 47
Goals of research 106

Health care 145

Intelligence 12
Interactive multimedia 156
Interactive training 156

Internal standards 101

Japan 70
Johns Hopkins 58

Leadership Qualities 8
Liabilities 140
Limitation of residency positions 45

Manual dexterity 27
Manual skills 27
Matching program 1
Molecular neurosurgery 145

Netherlands experience 33
Neurosurgeons in Japan 55
Neurosurgery 36, 40, 47, 93, 126
Neurosurgical manpower 30, 45
Neurosurgical research 111
Neurosurgical training 30, 43, 58, 73,
    79, 98
Non-academic hospital 79
Number of neurosurgeons 40

Objection of research training 111
Officers 22
Organ based programs 156
Organisation of surgical research 111

Pediatric neurosurgery 135
Performance criteria 19
Personality 12
Personnel recruitment 12
Perspective 89
Plastic trainers with integrated organs
    151
Portugal 43
Practice standards 126
Procedure in Great Britain 6
Professional training 126
Project financing 120

Profiles 22
Prominent Neurosurgeons 8

Radiosurgery 145
Realisation of research 120
Recruitment 45
Research foundations 120
Research rotation 106
Residency training 1
Resident experience 75
Resident suggestion 75
Resident training 33, 47

Selection of trainees 6
Selection process 1, 19
Simulation of situations 156
Skill assessment 27
Spain 43
Specific activities of neurosurgeons 55
Spine fellowship 130
Statistical prediction of needs 55
Stereotaxy 145
Structure 70
Subpecialisation 126
Subspeciality training 130, 135, 140
Success 8
Success indicators 12

Testing 22
Trainees 36
Training 93
Training contents 65
Training duration 65
Training program 70
Training systems in surgery 151

UEMS model 65
United States 30

Virtual-reality trainer 151

SpringerNeurosurgery

C. B. Ostertag, D. G. T. Thomas, A. Bosch, B. Linderoth, G. Broggi (eds.)

Advances in Stereotactic and Functional Neurosurgery 12

1997. 59 figures. X, 144 pages. Cloth DM 120,–, öS 840,–
Reduced price for subscribers to "Acta Neurochirurgica":
Cloth DM 108,–, öS 756,–. ISBN 3-211-82978-4
Acta Neurochirurgica, Supplement 68

The proceedings of the 12th Congress of the European Society for Stereotactic and Functional Neurosurgery in Milan contain selected contributions on surgery of Parkinson's disease, pain, psychosurgery, epilepsy, frameless stereotaxy, functional imaging, gene therapy and radiosurgery. The selection reflects the current status and progress in the field. The book is an update of the current methods and controversies and should serve those specialized in the field as a source of information and judgement. The foreword by Jens Haase unifies the views of both stereotactic and general neurosurgeons with great enthusiasm.

A. Mendelowitsch, H. Langemann, B. Alessandri, H. Landolt, O. Gratzl (eds.)

Clinical Aspects of Microdialysis

1996. 56 figures. VIII, 75 pages. Cloth DM 110,–, öS 770,–
Reduced price for subscribers to "Acta Neurochirurgica":
Cloth DM 99,–, öS 693,–. ISBN 3-211-82834-6
Acta Neurochirurgica, Supplement 67

This book contains papers presented at the First International Meeting on Clinical Aspects of Microdialysis in Basel, Switzerland. Microdialysis is a minimally invasive method which should have a future as a method for monitoring metabolic changes, e.g. during brain operations and neurosurgical intensive care, for glucose metabolism in diabetic patients, in neonates, etc. The meeting was organised to discuss the important step from experimental to clinical application of this method. It was the first meeting in the field to concentrate mainly on clinical aspects. The contributions represent the latest clinical and experimental findings and should be of great interest to clinicians and scientists.

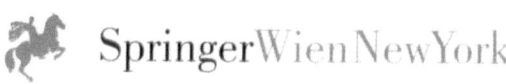

SpringerWienNewYork

Sachsenplatz 4-6, P.O.Box 89, A-1201 Wien, Fax +43-1-330 24 26, e-mail: order@springer.at, Internet: http://www.springer.at
New York, NY 10010, 175 Fifth Avenue • Heidelberger Platz 3, D-14197 Berlin • Tokyo 113, 3-13, Hongo 3-chome, Bunkyo-ku

Springer-Verlag
and the Environment

Springer-Verlag
and the Environment

WE AT SPRINGER-VERLAG FIRMLY BELIEVE THAT AN international science publisher has a special obligation to the environment, and our corporate policies consistently reflect this conviction.

WE ALSO EXPECT OUR BUSINESS PARTNERS - PRINTERS, paper mills, packaging manufacturers, etc. - to commit themselves to using environmentally friendly materials and production processes.

THE PAPER IN THIS BOOK IS MADE FROM LOW- OR NO-CHLORINE pulp and is acid free, in conformance with international standards for paper permanency.